A guide to the UK adult dental health survey 1998

The publication of this guide has been made possible by
financial support from the Department of Health and the
British Dental Association

A guide to the UK adult dental health survey 1998

N Nuttall
Senior Research Fellow, Dental Health Services Research Unit, University of Dundee

J G Steele
Senior Lecturer in Restorative Dentistry, University of Newcastle upon Tyne

J Nunn
Senior Lecturer and Honorary Consultant, University of Newcastle upon Tyne

C Pine
Reader and Honorary Consultant, University of Dundee

E Treasure
Professor of Dental Public Health, University of Wales

G Bradnock
Senior Lecturer in Dental Public Health, School of Dentistry, The University of Birmingham

J Morris
Lecturer in Dental Public Health, School of Dentistry, The University of Birmingham

M Kelly
Senior Social Survey Officer, Office for National Statistics, London

N B Pitts
Professor and Unit Director, Dental Health Services Research Unit, University of Dundee

D White
Lecturer, University of Birmingham

2001
Published by the British Dental Association
64 Wimpole Street, London, W1G 8YS

© British Dental Journal 2001

All rights reserved. No part of this publication may be reproduced, stored in a retrieval system, or transmitted in any form or by any means electronic, mechanical, photocopying, recording or otherwise, without either the permission of the publishers or a licence permitting restricted copying in the United Kingdom issued by the Copyright Licensing Agency Ltd, 90 Tottenham Court Road, London W1P 9HE

ISBN 0 904588 72 6

Printed and bound by Dennis Barber Graphics and Print,
Lowestoft, Suffolk

Foreword

The substance of this book is a collection of eight papers published in 2000 and 2001 in the *British Dental Journal*, reprinted as they appeared in the Journal. The aim is to provide an overview of the report of the 1998 UK Adult Dental Health Survey as a starting point for further discussion. However, it cannot replace the full report which remains the definitive account of the survey findings.

The series of Adult Dental Health studies are unique. They started in 1968 in England and Wales and in 1972 in Scotland. In 1978 the whole of the United Kingdom was surveyed at the same time, with oversampling in Wales and Scotland to enable separate reporting of findings in these countries along with England. With the 1998 survey we see the completion of the fourth survey and a description of oral health over the last 30 years. The surveys have all been undertaken by the Office of National Statistics (formerly Office of Population Censuses and Surveys) along with some of the dental schools of the United Kingdom. These have been the London Hospital Medical College Dental School in 1968, the dental schools of Universities of Dundee, Edinburgh & Glasgow in 1972, the dental schools of the Universities of Birmingham in 1978, 1988 and 1998; Newcastle upon Tyne in 1988 and 1998, and the dental schools of the Universities of Dundee and Wales in 1998. This combination of social survey researchers and dental epidemiologists allows for a strong study design and for considerable debate as to how the study should be carried out. In the latest survey there has been an even closer working relationship between the two sides of the team than before. This has led to an even greater emphasis on collaboration in design and in writing the report with the result that it has been possible to develop additional ways to spread the findings.

The aim of the surveys has been to report the oral health of a representative sample of the adult population and to make comparisons with previous surveys in order to describe changes that have occurred in oral health over the previous decade. The findings are relevant to everyone involved in dentistry in the United Kingdom. They give the big picture and identify trends. They allow any dentist to see their practice in the wider context and to think about and plan for the future.

The 1998 report is comprehensive, but it runs to 575 pages which does make it somewhat inaccessible to the practitioner and even the academic. Finding a specific piece of data may take some time and it can be quite hard to decide what the data mean. The nature of the report means that it is strictly an account of the data and as such does not allow for the data to be discussed and interpreted. Asking the question, 'What does this mean?' is not possible within the text. For these reasons a series of papers, summarising the findings of the survey and discussing their implications, were published. A key element of this series was to ask the question 'What do these results mean for practitioners and dental practice in the UK in the 21st century?'

Methodology

The survey was in two major parts. There was a questionnaire conducted by trained interviewers in people's own homes after which the participants were asked if they would consent to the second part; a dental examination by a survey dentist. The data gathering was undertaken by interviewers from the Social Survey Division of the Office for National Statistics and the Central Survey Unit in Northern Ireland. The dental examinations were undertaken by seventy-five dentists from the community dental service and health authorities specially trained for the purpose.

The questionnaire contained behavioural and attitudinal questions and, for the first time, a measure to investigate the impact that oral disease has on people's lives. However, the survey design remained comparable with the 1988 survey in order to ensure that valid comparisons with earlier surveys could be made. The sample was drawn by randomly selecting postcodes and then randomly selecting addresses. (In Northern Ireland a random selection of addresses was made.) The postcodes were stratified by region, socio-economic status and car ownership in order to ensure that the sample was representative. Proportionally larger samples were taken in Northern Ireland, Scotland and Wales so that valid results could be presented separately for each country. For any analysis of the UK the size of these samples was reduced by "weighting" them, to mirror their true proportion of the whole population.

The study design involved the development of the questionnaire and the clinical criteria for the dental examination. A pilot study was held to enable these instruments to be tested. Following revision of these, the final stage training and calibration exercises were held. Data were collected in the autumn of 1998. For the first time, data were collected directly onto laptop computers which removed the need for entering the data. This directly resulted in the much more rapid publication of the report. Following analysis, report writing and editing the full report was published early in 2000, a little over a year after the final data were collected.

The papers

The papers published here are intended to provide an overview of the results. Tooth loss, condition of the teeth and dental restorations are described in the first three papers.

The long term implications in the changes identified are discussed. The next two papers examine the interaction between factors associated with oral health and the impact of oral health on people. Both of these approaches are new to the 1998 survey and allow for a deeper understanding of the effects of oral disease. A further paper discusses the changing patterns of reported attendance and another considers dental attitudes and behaviours. Again both papers stress the implications for the future. Finally, there is a paper that describes the oral cleanliness and periodontal condition of the sample.

The opinions in the papers, as expressed in the discussion, are those of the individual authors. Other interpretations are possible and desirable. It is hoped that the publication of the papers in book form will stimulate discussion and improve access to the 1998 survey.

Acknowledgements

The study is complex to organise and depends on the goodwill as well as the hard work of many people. Subjects were required for the training, calibration and pilot studies. We especially thank those working at the ONS office and Patent Office in Newport, Gwent for assisting us. For the former some volunteered for more than one session. Dentists worked willingly to undertake the examinations mainly in the evenings and to help ensure adequate regional organisation. Interviewers were trained in dental terminology. We are very grateful to all these people for their willing help. We also gratefully acknowledge assistance with the funding of this publication from the Department of Health and the British Dental Association.

Disclaimer

This work was undertaken by a consortium comprising the Office for National Statistics and the Dental Schools of the Universities of Birmingham, Dundee, Newcastle and Wales who received funding from the United Kingdom Health Departments; the views expressed in this publication are those of the authors and not necessarily those of the Health Departments.

Contents

Total tooth loss in the United Kingdom in 1998 and implications for
the future   1

The condition of teeth in the UK in 1998 and implications for the
future   7

Dental restorations in adults in the UK in 1998 and implications for
the future   13

Factors associated with oral health: a multivariate analysis of results from the
1998 Adult Dental Health Survey   19

The impact of oral health on people in the UK in 1998   29

Dental attendance in 1998 and implications for the future   35

Dental attitudes and behaviours in 1998 and implications for the future   41

The oral cleanliness and periodontal health of UK adults in 1998   47

Index   55

Total tooth loss in the United Kingdom in 1998 and implications for the future

J. G. Steele,[1] E. Treasure,[2] N. B. Pitts,[3] J. Morris,[4] and G. Bradnock,[5]

The 1998 Adult Dental Health Survey, published this year, showed that the number of people without teeth should fall over the next three decades, to only 4% of the UK population. Patterns of tooth loss and retention are also changing. This article, the first of a series on the interpretation of the Adult Dental Health Survey, discusses the implications of these trends for dentistry.

At the time of the first national survey of adult dental health, which was held in 1968 and covered only England and Wales, over one third of the population (37%) had no natural teeth. Even amongst people aged 35–44 at that time, an edentulous mouth was a common finding (22%).[1] Times have changed. This paper will use data from the most recent United Kingdom Adult Dental Health Survey,[2] to describe the oral health of the nation in 1998. The data were also used to predict what is likely to happen over the next 20 or 30 years and these projections and their implications for the profession will be discussed.

For the purposes of this article, oral health is measured in very simple terms; the proportions of the population who have some natural teeth, the mean number of teeth they have and the proportions who have a 'functional' natural dentition. Although it is a crude measure of oral health, the proportion who have no natural teeth is both clear cut and important. However, as fewer people lose all of their teeth, its usefulness reduces, and other measures (such as the number of teeth and the proportion with a 'functional' natural dentition) may be necessary if an accurate indication of oral health is to be obtained from all patient groups. Data relating to these are also reported here in order to illustrate and discuss some of the important implications for dental practice from the findings of the survey.

The national surveys of Adult Dental Health have given a 10-yearly summary of the clinical condition of adults in the United Kingdom (England and Wales only in 1968, Scotland and Northern Ireland were surveyed later) on three previous occasions.[1–7] The fourth report in the series was published in March of 2000. For the 1998 survey 4,984 addresses were identified at which all resident adults aged over 16 years were asked to take part in the survey; 21% of households refused and no contact was made at 5%. In total, 6,204 adults were interviewed following which those with some teeth were asked to undergo a dental examination; 3,817 (72%) of those eligible agreed. A weighting system based on some of the interview responses of those who consented to be dentally examined and those who were interviewed but not dentally examined was used to reduce bias from non-response. The survey was carried out under the auspices of the Office of National Statistics together with the Universities of Birmingham, Dundee, Newcastle-upon-Tyne and Wales.

Who had no natural teeth at all in 1998?

The irreversible nature of the two main destructive dental diseases (caries and periodontal disease) dictate that age is always likely to be a principal factor associated with total tooth loss. Figure 1 shows the proportion who do and do not have teeth, plotted against age. Although 87% of all adults had some natural teeth, up to the age of 45 the figure was almost 100%, while over the age of 54 being edentate was still a relatively common occurrence. Amongst people aged 75 and over, those without natural teeth were still in the majority (58%). Nevertheless, the retention of some natural teeth is now sufficiently common that, amongst the 'younger-old' population nearly two thirds (64%) of the 65–74 year age group and more than half of all of the people of 'pensionable' age in the UK (54%) now have at least a few natural teeth. Over the age of 44 though, the age related difference in the proportion of the population without any teeth was quite marked. Perhaps it is of relevance that the population below this age in 1998 had had an entire lifetime of the National Health Service (assuming they have been residents throughout), but that this was not the case for those aged 50 or over in 1998 (Fig. 1).

Social class, in combination with gender, was also associated with having no teeth. Social class differences in total tooth loss were much greater among men than women and this was particularly noticeable amongst older men in comparison with older women (Fig. 2). It is difficult to be sure why older men from non-manual backgrounds were more likely to have teeth than those from manual working backgrounds, while women did not appear to show the same social class difference. When multivariate analyses were undertaken to control for the effects of confounding variables such as age, marital status and various others, the association with gender disappeared. The

[1]Senior Lecturer in Restorative Dentistry, University of Newcastle upon Tyne, [2]Professor of Dental Public Health, University of Wales, [3]Professor and Unit Director, Dental Health Services Research Unit, University of Dundee, [4]Lecturer in Dental Public Health and Senior Lecturer in Dental Public Health, [5]The University of Birmingham
*Correspondence to: Dr J.G.Steele, Dental School, Framlington Place, Newcastle upon Tyne, NE2 4BW
email: j.g.steele@ncl.ac.uk
REFEREED PAPER
Received 12.06.00; Accepted 31.07.00
© British Dental Journal 2000; 189: 598–603

In brief
- In 1998, 87% of all adults had natural teeth
- By 2028 it should be about 96%
- A small but varied group of people will continue to become edentulous
- The replacement of missing teeth in partial dentitions will continue to be very common for the foreseeable future

A guide to the UK adult dental health survey 1998

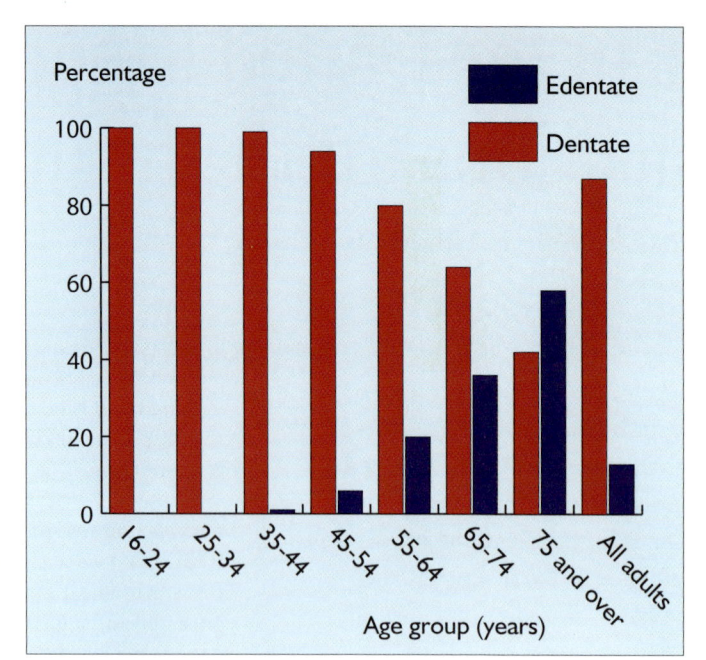

Fig. 1 Dental status by age in the United Kingdom in 1998

differences observed according to gender may be accounted for by other factors, such as marital status. The role of social class (which was still significant in the multivariate analysis) perhaps suggests that differences arise from social values associated with appearance, and the contribution, or otherwise, made to appearance by natural teeth in older people (Fig. 2).

Are there still regional differences in total tooth loss?

The first Adult Dental Health survey in 1968 showed the profound differences in various measures of oral health between the North and South of England.[1] Subsequent surveys undertaken in 1972 and 1979 clearly showed that this extended to Scotland and Northern Ireland as well.[5,6] The 1998 survey has found these differences persist in many instances (Fig. 3). The area with the highest proportion of the population with some natural teeth was the South of England where 90% of the population (93% of men and 88% of women) was dentate. The rest of the country lagged some way behind with the lowest proportion of adults with some natural teeth being in Scotland (83%).

There are differences in the social class structure of the regions and countries of the United Kingdom that potentially could account for the differences between them. However, the differences persist to some extent, even between similar social class groups in different parts of the United Kingdom, suggesting that there has been a cultural dimension to the pattern of total tooth loss around the country. Taking all of the factors together produces quite profound differences; women from an unskilled manual background living in Scotland (amongst whom 36% were edentate), were 12 times more likely to have no teeth at all, than men from a non-manual background in the south of England (3% edentate). Generally speaking, women from unskilled working backgrounds were the population group with the lowest proportion of people with some natural teeth.

In terms of the geographical variation it is really the South of England which is at variance from most of the rest of the country. Overall, 90% of people in the South of England were dentate, but the proportions in the other areas were relatively similar (83–86%), with only Northern Ireland approaching the South of England in terms of the proportion with teeth (88%). Despite these differences within the United Kingdom, many of the cases where there are no natural teeth actually reflect what happened many years ago. All areas of the country are seeing a similar rapid reduction in the prevalence of edentulousness, but in crude

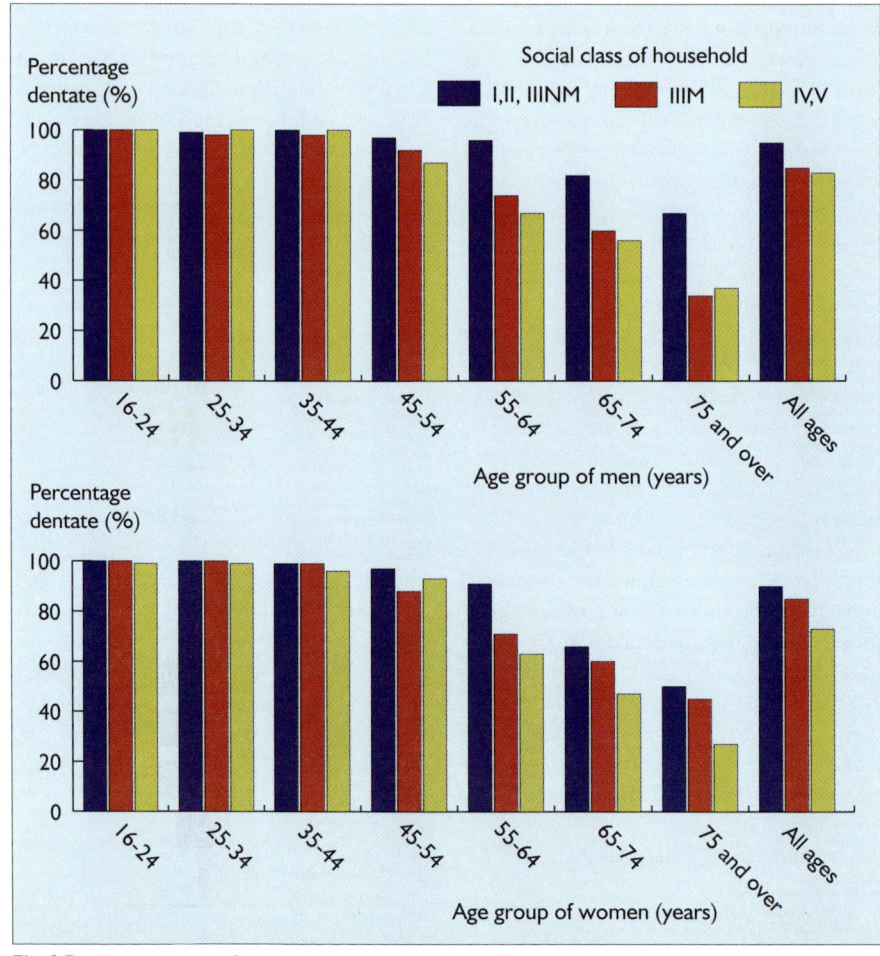

Fig. 2 Data: percentage dentate by age and social class of head of household as defined by occupation in the United Kingdom in 1998. Data for men and women are presented separately.

Total tooth loss

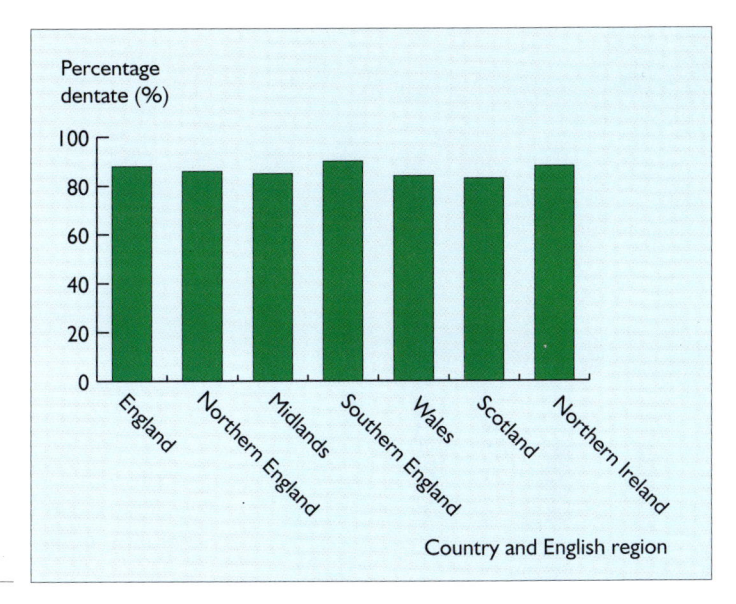

Fig. 3 Percentage dentate by home country and English regions

terms the rest of country reached the point in 1998 which the South of England had already reached at the last survey in 1988, so the South of England is further forward in the process. The patterns we see now therefore may not reflect the current pattern in the incidence (new cases) of total tooth loss. This leads us on to the next question, which relates to these new cases of total tooth loss.

Who became edentate in the 1990s?

Although the overall prevalence of total tooth loss has fallen sharply over recent decades, there are still people who are becoming edentulous. These people are important because, although their numbers are small, they are potentially quite difficult to manage clinically.

Only 96 people out of over 6,000 who were interviewed had lost all of their teeth in the 10 years preceding the survey.[1] This represents between 1% and 2% of the sample. All age categories were represented, including one 18-year-old. Twenty-six people aged less than 55 in 1998 had lost all of their teeth sometime in the preceding 10 years, but most were aged 55 years or over at the time of the survey. In contrast to the historical distribution of edentulousness, the social and geographical distribution of these people was rather even, with no social groups or parts of the country being obviously more affected than others. With so few people involved it would have been difficult to identify subtle trends with confidence, but no obvious differences emerged.

How and why did they lose their teeth?

The pattern of loss of the last teeth has changed markedly. People who became edentulous in the period tended to have fewer teeth removed at their final clearance than has been the case in the past. In 1968 two-thirds of people who had lost all of their teeth had had 12 or more teeth removed at their final clearance, 10 years later this had dropped to one-half, by 1998 it was only one-quarter. The fact that fewer teeth are now being removed at final clearance probably reflects a combination of factors, such as a reduction in the number of people who have devastating amounts of oral disease and perhaps also a greater determination among patients and their dentists to retain some natural teeth for as long as possible.

Those who lost their teeth in the preceding 10 years were asked what they thought

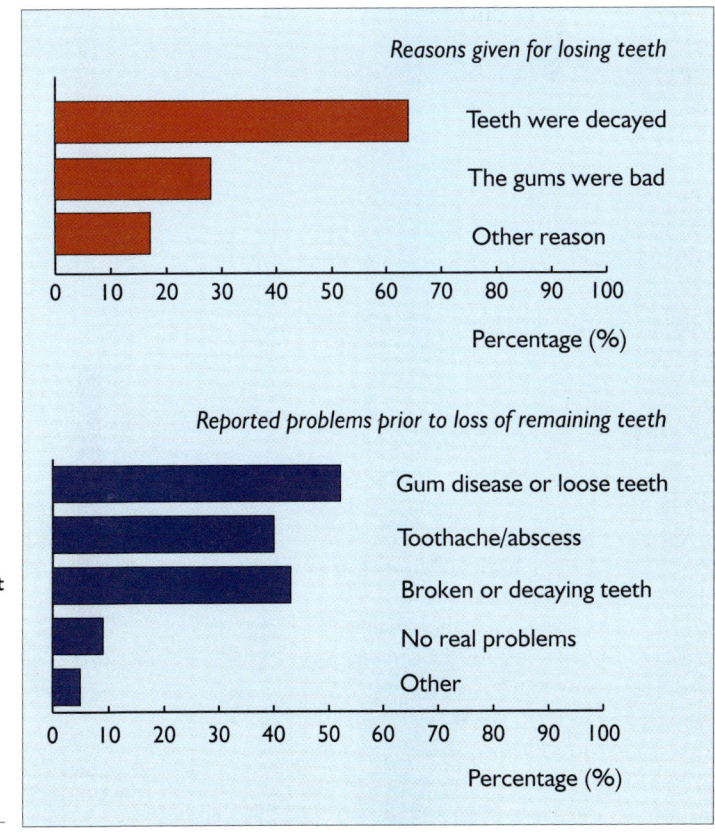

Fig. 4 Reasons for losing the last remaining teeth and reported problems prior to loss among people who had become edentulous in the previous 10 years

the reason for loss of their last remaining teeth was and what problems they had prior to losing them (Fig. 4). Decayed teeth was the most frequently cited cause for final clearance (in 64% of cases) and 28% said it was caused by bad gums. However, when asked what problems they had experienced just prior to having all their teeth taken out, over a half mentioned having had some gum problems or loose teeth. Less than one in ten people said they had no real dental problems prior to the loss of the last of their teeth.

What do we expect the level of total tooth loss to be in future?

According to the projections, which used the same methods as were used successfully for the 1988 survey, it is unlikely that we will reach a stage where edentulousness disappears completely from the population. The trend has been evident now since the first survey in England and Wales in 1968, and can be seen clearly in Figure 5. Projections using data from 1988 and 1998 show that

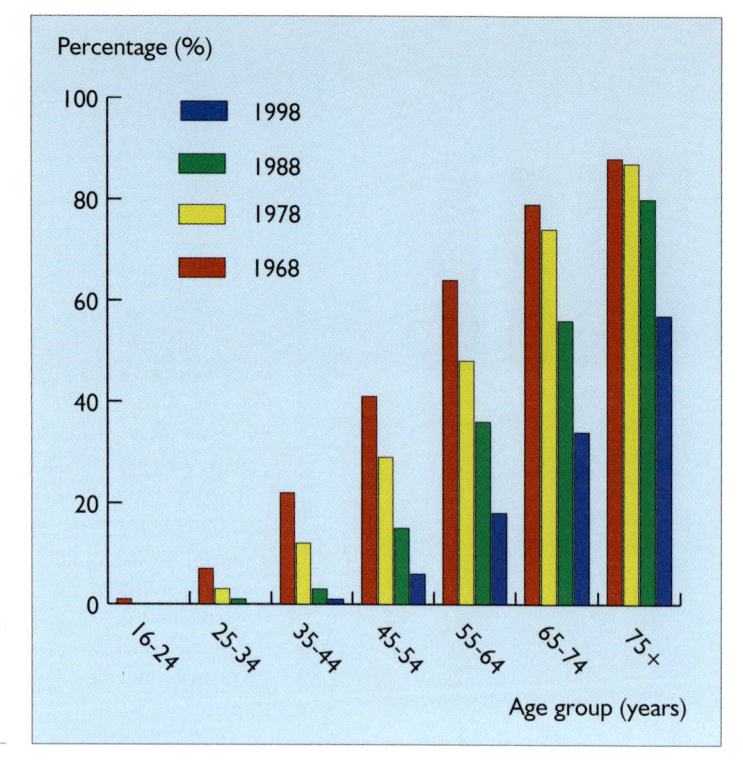

A guide to the UK adult dental health survey 1998

Fig. 5 Trends in the percentage of adults without natural teeth, 1968-1998, the UK trends are very similar

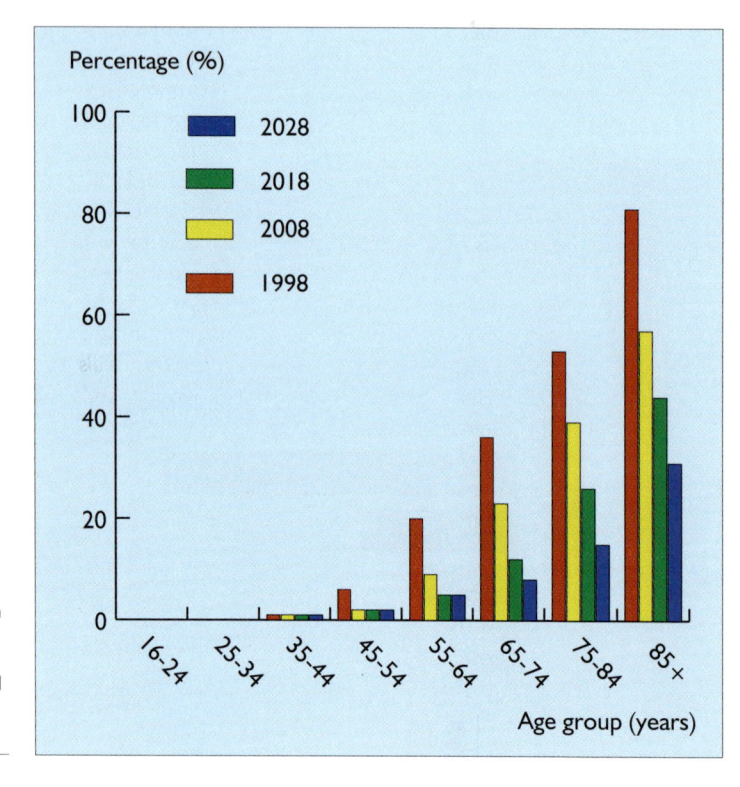

Fig. 6 Projections of future trends in the percentage of UK adults without natural teeth, 1998-2028

the proportion of people with no teeth at all is expected to drop to 8% in 2008 and to 5% by 2018 (Fig. 6). It does not show any sign of disappearing completely because a small number of new cases continue to arise, and this incidence was only slightly lower in the last decade than it was in the previous one. Although these people will mostly be old, (over the age of 75 years) the data on recent cases of total tooth loss suggest that there will still be a reasonable proportion of them in late middle age, perhaps particularly those who suffer from advanced periodontal disease (half of them reported gum disease or loose teeth prior to losing the last of their teeth). If the recent pattern of new cases continues they will be more evenly distributed on the social and geographical spectrum than the current prevalence data suggest (Figs 5 and 6).

Do the people who have teeth have more of them than they used to?
Retaining natural teeth is all very well, but is only likely to be a major benefit if enough of them are retained to allow better function than would be the case without them.

In fact, the number of teeth which people have has also increased over recent years. The average number of teeth (amongst people with teeth) was 24.8, but this was obviously highest among the younger groups, reducing quite sharply among the oldest. This compares with 23.1 teeth among dentate people 20 years ago. Bearing in mind that the proportion of people with teeth has increased substantially in that time, the real increase in the total number of teeth in the country will have been much greater (Fig. 7).

The number of teeth varied to some extent according to gender, social class and geography, but the factor which appeared to make the biggest impact was whether or not people said that they went to the dentist for regular check-ups. The difference between 'check-up' attenders and people who said they only attended when they had trouble was small in the younger age groups. However as age increased, and the cumulative effects of untreated disease were felt, a considerable gulf opened up. Among 55–64 year olds the difference between the two groups was an average of six teeth. In terms of tooth retention, dental attendance does appear to be of substantial benefit over the course of a lifetime (Fig. 8).

Just as the retention of some teeth is increasing, so is the retention of a 'functional dentition'. The proportion of people with 21 or more teeth is used as a way of recording a 'functional dentition'. Although the figure is essentially arbitrary, the relevance of the 21 tooth threshold is backed up by evidence relating to diet and comfort.[8-11] Altering the figure to '22 or more' or '20 or more' teeth would make relatively little difference, but it is around this point or above that people tend to experience dietary freedom and be able to rely on natural teeth without dentures for comfortable function. In this survey it represented a sharp cut-off point for partial denture wearing (Fig. 9).

Over 72% of all adults had 21 or more natural teeth in 1998, but the figures amongst older adults are much lower; only 10% of all people aged 75 or over had 21 or more teeth. Projecting forwards from these

Total tooth loss

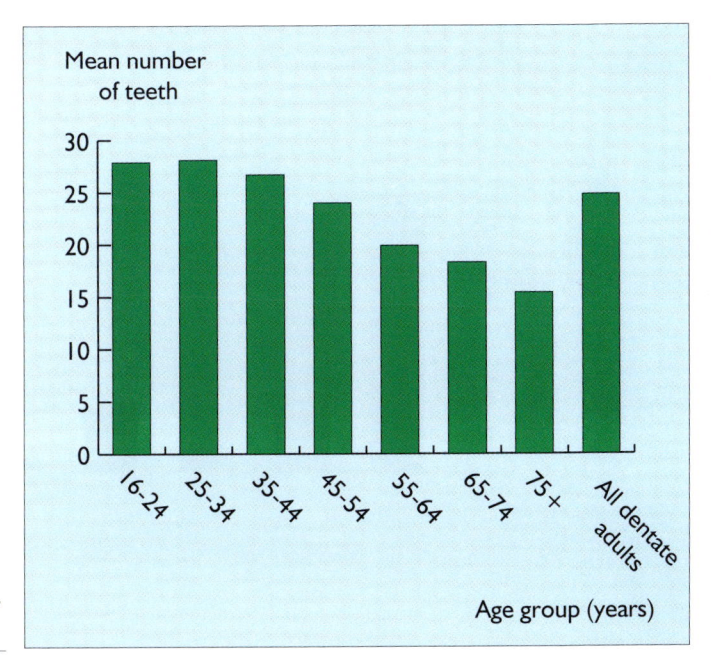

Fig. 7 Mean number of teeth by age

data, around 90% of 16–74 year olds should have a natural dentition of 21 or more teeth by 2018, but the figure will be lower for older people. The trend is certainly towards retaining a functional dentition into old age, although perhaps not for an entire lifetime. It will be a very long time indeed though before the proportion of the population with 21 or more teeth approaches 100%. A combination of natural teeth and dentures will still be as common as ever for the next couple of decades at least, and the management of this situation, particularly amongst older adults, will be a very important issue for dentists for many years to come. This brings us on to the next question.

What does the declining incidence of edentulousness and the increase in the number of people with a functional natural dentition imply for the profession in the future?

It is easy to assume that, with the proportion of United Kingdom adults who are edentate decreasing to around only 5% over the next 20 years, the need for skills in complete denture prosthodontics will diminish. The reality is likely to be somewhat more complex. The predicted 5% of the adult population in 2018 may not sound like a lot, but it still accounts for a couple of million adults, and a similar number of sets of complete dentures in circulation. In the past, undergraduate students developed skills in prosthodontics which they had ample opportunity to refine and consolidate in dental practice. Nowadays, with perhaps four or five million edentate adults, many dental schools are already finding it difficult to identify appropriate undergraduate teaching material. In future, teaching hospitals are likely to find cases even more difficult to come by and many dentists in practice are likely to see too few cases to maintain their skills and confidence, let alone to develop them.

The increasing complexity of many such cases, and perhaps also the increasing reluctance of our patients to become one of the small proportion of edentate people (data from the survey also supports this attitudinal trend), may make a large number of cases very challenging to manage. One likely outcome is that many dentists may feel uncomfortable about treating such patients and their management may be transferred to the minority of dentists who have specific expertise or training in this area of dental care. We may also expect the use of implant technology to continue to develop.

For their part, many undergraduate schools have already changed their training strategy, but further alterations may need to be made in this important area of dentistry in order to deal with this evolving situation. For dentists who have finished their undergraduate training and are starting out in their careers, skills in complete denture prosthodontics may turn out to be more useful than it may seem from the bald statistics presented in the report, but only for those who are prepared to develop them to a high level.

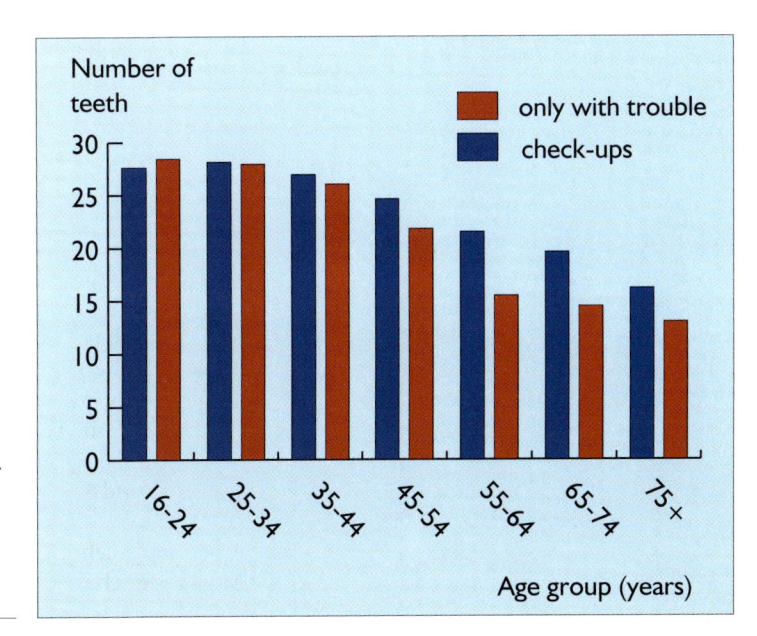

Fig. 8 Differences in the number of teeth by age according to reported attendance status

A guide to the UK adult dental health survey 1998

These data are also of enormous relevance to the current debate about the training of 'denturists'. Whilst we have no wish to enter this particular argument here, whether you support or reject the potential introduction of trained denturists, there is no doubt that this changing environment, including the potential alterations in undergraduate and postgraduate training and in referral patterns, ought to be major considerations.

There have been clear improvements in the proportion of the population achieving the '21 or more teeth' threshold, but it will be a long time before a majority of older people will be able to function without the need for some sort of prosthesis to fill the gaps left by lost teeth. Appropriate management of older dentate people will continue to involve managing depleted dentitions with the various prosthodontic, restorative and preventive skills that this entails. Indeed, given the slowing of the pace of the transition to total tooth loss and the apparent increase in demands for tooth preservation, these skills are likely to see plenty of scope for improvement.

Are there any management issues for the individual patient?

Even if many practitioners choose to refer their complete denture patients for the construction of dentures, dental disease in the earlier stages of the pathway to total tooth loss will still need to be managed by the general dentist. The new cases could arise anywhere in the country, and although the overall incidence will be very low, complete tooth loss may affect anybody. However, the risk of losing all teeth should be obvious some time before the last teeth are removed. People taking part in the survey in 1998 were asked how upset they were at losing the last of their teeth. The resulting data suggest that people who lose the last of their teeth in years to come may be rather reluctant to do so. People who expected to lose their teeth were significantly less likely to be upset about the process than those for whom it was a surprise. If the candidates for total tooth loss can be identified early, good communication and sensible long-term planning may save a great deal of heartache later on.

How quickly will these changes occur?

It will take time for the oldest cohort of people, who have been edentate for many years, to be lost completely from the population, and all of the other trends are gradual. They will however be very apparent within just a part of a practising lifetime.

This article has been refereed under the British Dental Journal reviewing process. Full details of sample numbers and the criteria for the clinical examinations can be found in the survey report. We would like to acknowledge the work of Alison Walker, Maureen Kelly and other staff of the Office for National Statistics.
This work was undertaken by a consortium comprising the Office for National Statistics and the Dental Schools of the Universities of Birmingham, Dundee, Newcastle and Wales who received funding from the United Kingdom Health Departments; the views expressed in this publication are those of the authors and not necessarily those of the Health Departments nor of the other members of the consortium.

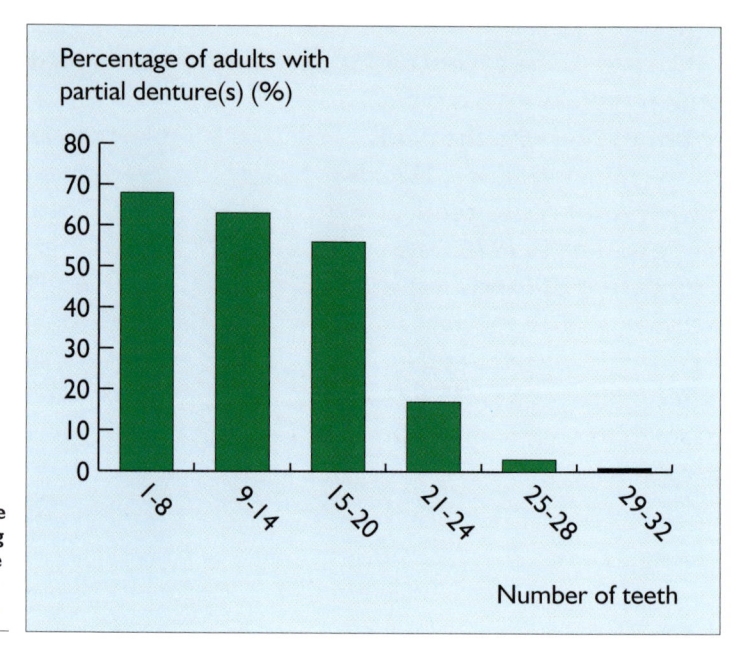

Fig. 9 Percentage of adults wearing a partial denture according to the number of teeth

1. Gray P G, Todd J E, Slack G L, Bulman J S. *Adult Dental Health in England and Wales in 1968.* London: TSO, 2000
2. Kelly M, Steele J G, Nuttall N, Bradnock G, Morris J, Nunn J et al. *Adult Dental Health Survey: Oral health in the United Kingdom 1998.* London: TSO, 1970
3. Todd J E, Walker A M. *Adult dental health. Volume 2: United Kingdom 1978.* London: HMSO, 1982.
4. Todd J E, Walker A M. *Adult Dental Health. Volume 1: England and Wales.* London: HMSO 1980.
5. Todd J E, Whitworth A. *Adult Dental Health in Scotland 1972.* London: HMSO, 1974.
6. Todd J E, Lader D. *Adult Dental Health 1988. United Kingdom.* London: HMSO, 1991.
7. Rhodes J R, Haire T H. *Adult dental health survey Northern Ireland 1979.* Belfast: HMSO, 1979.
8. Steele J G, Sheiham A, Marcenes W, Walls A W G. *National Diet and Nutrition Survey: people aged 65 and over Volume 2: Report of the oral health survey.* London: TSO 1998.
9. Agerberg G, Carlsson G E. Chewing ability in relation to dental and general health. *Acta Odont Scand* 1981; **39:** 147-153.
10. Witter D J, Cramwinckel A B, Van Rossum G M J M, Kayser A F. Shortened dental arches and masticatory ability. *J Dent* 1990; **18:**185-189.
11. Aukes J N S C, Kayser A F, Felling A J A. The subjective experience of mastication in subjects with shortened dental arches. *J Oral Rehabil* 1988; **15:** 321-324.

The condition of teeth in the UK in 1998 and implications for the future

J. Nunn,[1] J. Morris,[2] C. Pine,[3] N. B. Pitts,[4] G. Bradnock,[5] and J. Steele,[6]

The latest of the decennial surveys of the United Kingdom was undertaken in 1998 by the Office of National Statistics in collaboration with the dental schools of the Universities of Birmingham, Dundee, Newcastle and Wales. Dentate adults in 1998 have fewer missing teeth and more sound and untreated teeth on average than in 1978. The average number of decayed teeth has dropped significantly from 1.9 in 1978 to 1.1 in 1998. The average number of filled teeth has remained fairly constant over the same time but its distribution has changed quite markedly towards older adults having more filled teeth than people of a similar age in the past whilst the reverse is true for younger adults. The overall trends are encouraging, but there is a need to review the way disease is managed in adults in the United Kingdom.

In brief
- Among young adults, dental caries predominantly affected the first and second premolars of 16-24 year olds. Most of these teeth were not fissure sealed.
- The bulk of filled teeth is now amongst older adults, whilst the number in young adults is falling
- 11% of adults had tooth wear on anterior teeth which was rated as moderate or worse.
- Decay of root surfaces was uncommon in younger adults, but amongst adults aged 65 years and over an average of 10.6 teeth were vulnerable, and a third had root caries lesions.

In most of the westernised countries that undertake oral health surveys, oral health has generally improved. Even those countries which have had very high levels of disease have shown reductions in dental disease experience, often most apparent in the younger age groups.[1,2] On the whole though, people have more teeth than they had in the past and more of them are disease-free.[3–5]

The national surveys of Adult Dental Health have given a 10-yearly summary of the clinical condition of adults in the United Kingdom on three previous occasions. The fourth report in the series was published in March of 2000.[6] For the 1998 survey 4,984 addresses were identified at which all adults over 16 in residence were asked to take part in the survey; 21% of households refused and no contact was made at 5% of them. In total, 6,204 adults were interviewed following which those with some teeth were asked to undergo a dental examination; 3,817 (72%) of those eligible agreed. A weighting system based on some of the interview responses of those who consented to be dentally examined and those who were interviewed but not dentally examined was used to reduce bias from non-response.[6] The survey was carried out under the auspices of the Office of National Statistics together with the Universities of Birmingham, Dundee, Newcastle-upon-Tyne and Wales.

The clinical examinations collected information about the state of the teeth and restorations as well as information on spacing and how this is restored. It was felt important to include, for the first time, an assessment of visual caries (dentine involvement but not cavitated lesions) as well as lesions that had proceeded to cavitation. In younger populations especially, the former is an important marker of disease typically requiring restorative intervention. Also for the first time, tooth wear was measured. This article looks at the condition of teeth in the United Kingdom.

Has the overall condition of teeth changed since 1978?
Figure 1 shows that the number of teeth among dentate adults without signs of disease or treatment has increased since 1978

[1]*Senior Lecturer, Honorary Consultant, University of Newcastle upon Tyne;* [2]*Lecturer, University of Birmingham;* [3]*Reader, Honorary Consultant, University of Dundee;* [4]*Director, Dental Health Services Research Unit, University of Dundee;* [5]*Senior Lecturer, University of Birmingham;* [6]*Senior Lecturer, University of Newcastle upon Tyne*
Correspondence to: Dr June Nunn, Department of Child Dental Health, Dental School, Framlington Place, Newcastle upon Tyne NE2 4BW
email: J.H.Nunn@ncl.ac.uk
Refereed Paper
Received 12.06.00; Accepted 03.07.00
© *British Dental Journal* 2000; **189:** 639–644

Table 1	The mean number of teeth restored, otherwise sound by age 1978–1998 (1998 data is based on 1988 criteria)		
Dentate adults			*United Kingdom*
Age group (years)	1978	1988	1998
All	8.1	8.4	8.1
16–24	8.0	5.5	2.9
25–34	9.8	10.0	7.4
35–44	8.9	11.1	10.1
45–54	7.1	9.6	11.1
55–64	4.8	7.1	9.0
65–74	4.8	5.7	8.2
75 and over	4.8	3.7	6.5

A guide to the UK adult dental health survey 1998

Fig. 1 The mean number of teeth in each condition, 1978–98:
(a) missing, (b) decayed or unsound, (c) restored, otherwise sound,
(d) sound and untreated (1998 data is based on 1988 criteria)

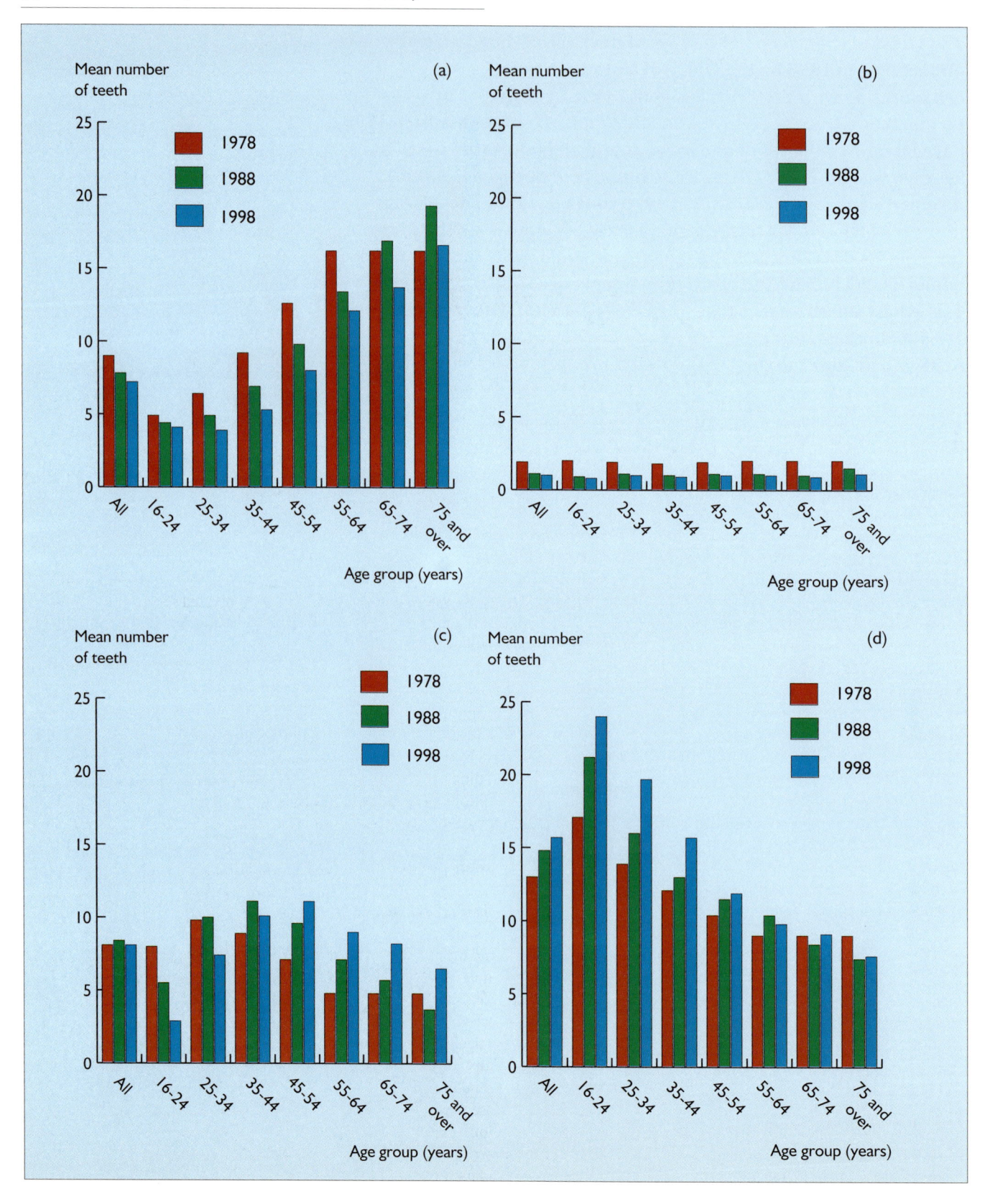

The condition of teeth

from 13 sound and untreated teeth on average to 15.7 in 1998. Over the same period the number of filled teeth has stayed much the same at around 8.1 teeth between 1978 and 1998 but the number of teeth which are either decayed or missing has dropped, in the case of untreated decay by almost a half, over the last 20 years.

However, this conceals an important age trend. Filled teeth have declined markedly among young adults but increased among older adults (Table 1). Dentate adults aged 16–24 had an average of 2.9 filled teeth in 1998 compared with 8.0 in 1978. Among dentate adults aged over 45 the average number of filled teeth in 1998 had risen by at least 50% of the average in 1978. Is this a sign of unnecessary dental treatment in the past among the older age groups? We think not; the average number of sound and untreated teeth among older dentate adults has not decreased as restorative treatment has increased. What has decreased among this group is the number of decayed and the number of missing teeth. This suggests that the increased experience of restorative dental treatment among the elderly is by and large reflected by a lessening experience of tooth loss. However, with increasing age, more and more teeth become involved in the restorative cycle, particularly in middle age. For adults aged over 55 years, a significant disability may be imposed by the extraction of diseased teeth.

What is the type and extent of dental caries among dentate adults in the United Kingdom?

In previous national dental surveys the assessment of dental decay included a measurement of cavitated lesions and severely broken down teeth only. In the 1998 survey, in addition to these more advanced signs of decay an assessment of visual decay (the stage of the caries process where there is demineralisation but not cavitation) was included to give a more realistic assessment of the current prevalence of dental decay.

Overall 24% of dentate adults had visual primary caries, 22% primary cavitated caries and 8% had recurrent cavitated caries (Fig. 2).

Whilst dental intervention, sealants, dietary messages, plaque control, and minimal restorations, would seem to be appropriate, given what happens to the dental health of the cohorts as they age, it need not necessarily be given by dentists. Indeed, in the light of the likely work required, it may not need to be. The advent of professions complementary to dentistry (PCDs) within dental practice may in future lead to a more cost-effective skill mix within primary care dentistry to enable such a strategy to be adopted, notwithstanding the evolving nature of clinical conditions that will need to be managed over the next few decades.

Which teeth have been affected by caries?

Figure 3 shows the distribution of dental caries (cavitated lesions affecting dentine) and its treatment around the mouth of dentate adults. Overall, molars were the teeth most affected by disease, with 85% of them either missing, decayed, unsound or restored. This was particularly marked for the youngest age group, 16–24 year-olds, where the first and second molar teeth bear the brunt of the disease experience. Apart from a small proportion of restorations in teeth that are more anterior in the arch, and the loss of first premolars for orthodontic purposes, about one third of first permanent molars are restored and just over one tenth have untreated decay.

The distribution of different conditions around the mouth shows that the majority of disease experienced in the youngest age group and for successive cohorts is concentrated in first and second molar teeth.[6] The application of sealants to these teeth could dramatically alter the overall disease experience both now and in the future. As it is, a significant number of teeth will require maintenance and re-maintenance for years to come. Yet fissure sealants were only found in 23% of this age group.

The survey reports that there is almost 50% less decay in those who attend for regular dental check-ups than those who only go to a dentist when they have trouble with their teeth.[6] However, it is disturbing that over one third of regular attenders have some form of decay, albeit largely primary, visual decay. Of concern is the relatively high proportion of 16–24 year-olds who have decay; half have some primary decay, a third of which is visual, a fifth cavitated and 6% have unrestorable teeth. Whilst these young people have, until recently, had access to dental to care in either general dental

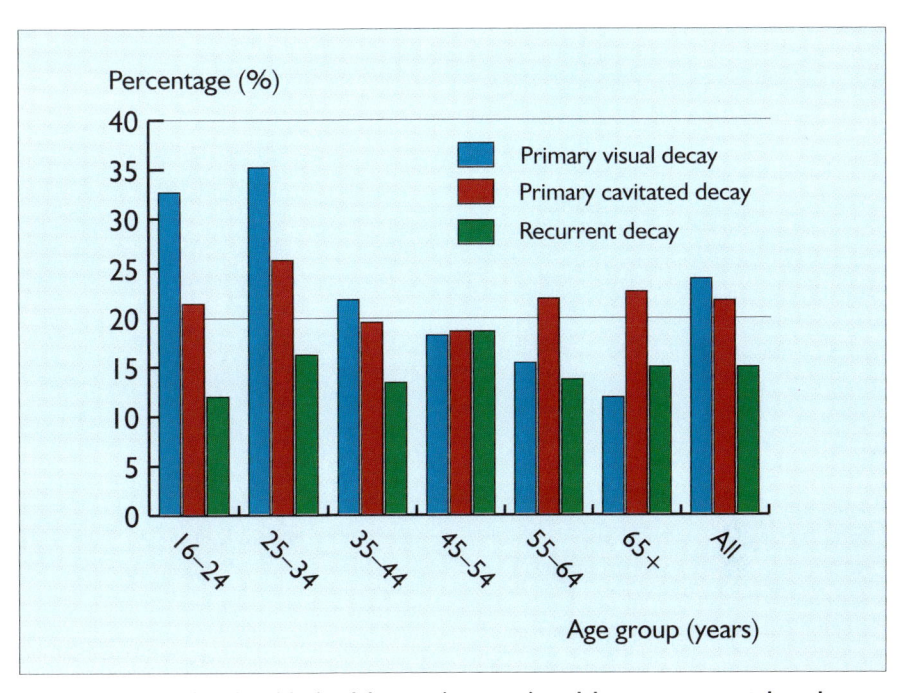

Fig. 2 Proportion of adults with visual decay, primary cavitated decay or recurrent decay by age

A guide to the UK adult dental health survey 1998

practice or the community dental service, only 49% of this age group reported visiting a dentist regularly. Forty eight per cent of the 16–24-year-olds, reported less frequent attendance than five years ago.[6]

Although it is up to the individual as to whether they visit a dentist, the dental service could be seen to be failing in one of its objectives, of encouraging routine dental care, when so many of its regular patients do not maintain this attendance pattern. A significant proportion of the population seemingly does not receive regular care at all. What role should the dental profession play in this?

Root caries
One of the concerns in the dental profession is the propensity for an increase in the prevalence and incidence of root caries given the changing age profile of the population and the increasing retention of natural teeth into old age. Linked with this are the age-associated changes in the periodontal tissues such that vulnerable root surfaces are exposed to the oral environment and thus, potentially, the caries process.

Two thirds of all adults had at least one tooth with a root surface which was vulnerable to decay (either exposed, worn, decayed or filled), and on average 6.4 teeth were in this condition. However, the pattern was not uniform with only 1.2 vulnerable teeth in younger adults compared with 10.6 in adults aged 65 years and over. This represents well over half of the teeth present at this age. Amongst the 29% of older adults (65+) who had root caries, on average 2.3 teeth were affected. By contrast, 54% of older adults had some caries around the crown of the tooth (often recurrent around existing restorations), and the number of teeth affected was very similar to that for roots (2.2). The prevalence of caries on root surfaces is approaching that for coronal caries in older people. The majority of decay affecting roots was active decay (9% of vulnerable surfaces), as opposed to arrested (2%), recurrent (1%) or unrestorable (3%) decay.

On the basis of these data, root caries is not likely to be a huge public health problem in younger age groups. However, in older age groups a significant proportion of the caries burden falls on the exposed roots. Most of

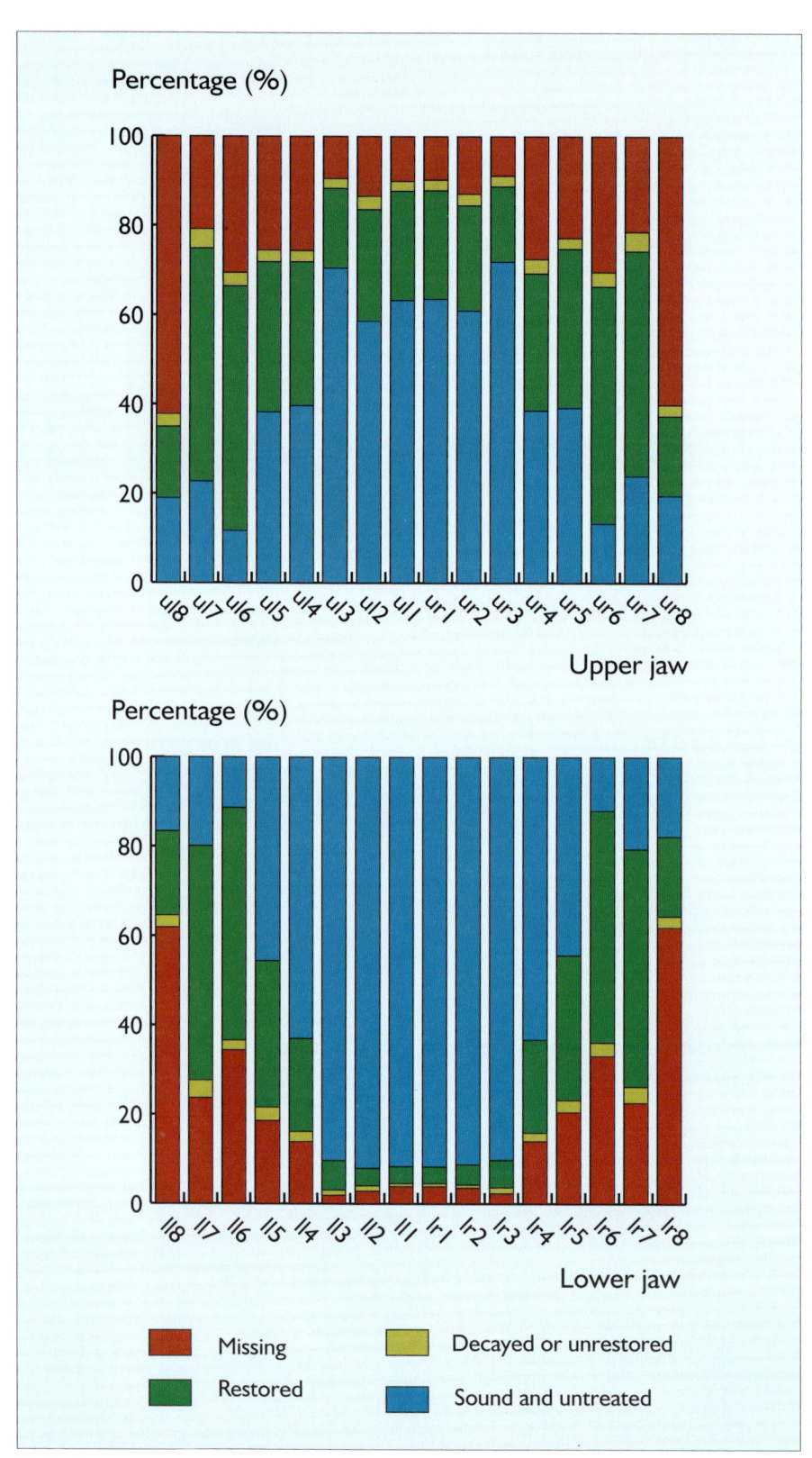

Fig. 3 Distribution of tooth conditions around the mouth

The condition of teeth

Table 2: Amount and degree of tooth wear by age, gender, country, English region, social class of head of household, and usual reason for dental attendance

Dentate adults United Kingdom

	Mean proportion of teeth with:			Base
	Any tooth wear	Some moderate wear	Some severe wear	
All	34	3	0	3817
Age				
16–24	12	0	0	491
25–34	24	1	0	854
35–44	29	2	0	781
45–54	41	4	0	746
55–64	49	5	0	461
65 and over	58	9	2	484
Gender				
Men	40	4	1	1745
Women	28	2	0	2072
Country				
England	34	3	0	2186
Wales	37	4	0	502
Scotland	31	2	0	668
Northern Ireland	37	2	0	461
English region				
North	37	4	1	617
Midlands	33	2	0	495
South	32	3	0	1074
Social class of head of household				
I, II, IIINM	34	2	0	1926
IIIM	37	4	0	1025
IV, V	34	4	0	625
Usual reason for dental attendance				
Regular check-up	34	3	0	2400
Occasional check-up	30	2	0	408
Only with trouble	37	4	1	10003

the root caries found in this survey related to new lesions. This is in contrast to the rather higher proportion (around a third) of decay in the crowns of the teeth which was recurrent around existing restorations. Some of the interventions required to treat the root decay in older adults will certainly be operative, but much of it may be able to be dealt with more simply. The scope for preventive care is considerable. A concerted preventive strategy for the younger cohorts of adults who are still disease free, and for the older adults at greatest risk of root caries may make an impact. This may be another area where the PCDs have a role to play.

Less disease — but are they wearing away?
To an extent, tooth wear is part of the normal ageing process of the dentition. When it is excessive, such that the longevity of the tooth is threatened, it becomes a clinical concern. Alongside this of course are considerations of the patient-driven concerns about poor aesthetics, sensitivity and with increasingly severe wear, function.

- The clinical examination was confined to the palatal, labial and incisal surfaces of the six upper anterior teeth, and the worst affected surface of the lower anterior teeth. These surfaces were selected on the basis of evidence from previous surveys[7,8] as being the ones most likely to be affected if wear was present elsewhere in the mouth.

The data were categorized as follows for the purpose of presentation:

- Any tooth wear, excluding that confined only to enamel
- Moderate wear — involving more extensive exposure of dentine
- Severe wear — complete enamel loss with exposure of pulp or secondary dentine.

Two thirds of all adults had some wear into dentine on anterior teeth. For 11% of adults the wear was moderate (extensive involvement of dentine) and 1% had severe wear. As with most other dental conditions, the prevalence of tooth wear did increase with age: a third of the youngest adults had some evidence of tooth wear on anterior

A guide to the UK adult dental health survey 1998

teeth compared with 89% of those aged 65 years and over. There were no significant differences in the prevalence of any tooth wear recorded between people from different social classes or different attendance patterns, but more males than females had some tooth wear, especially severe tooth wear. Scottish adults were least likely to have any tooth wear compared with the other countries of the UK. There were little inter-regional differences for tooth wear but those adults living in the Midlands had less moderate tooth wear (7%) than did adults living in the north or the south (12%) of England. Geographical differences should be interpreted with some caution though because of the possibility of inter-examiner variability.

Contrasting these data with that from the oldest age group in the 1993 UK children's dental health survey,[9] (the young people who would therefore be included in the 16–24-year-old group in the 1998 adult survey), there was a similar amount of tooth wear in both groups; in the children's dental health survey, 2% of the older children were recorded as having wear into dentine/pulp, comparable to the moderate/severe categories in this study — in 1998, 1% of 16–24-year-olds had moderate tooth wear (Table 2).

It is encouraging to note that there has apparently been virtually no increase in the amount of wear in young peoples' teeth over the past few years; the children's dental health survey[9] showed quite a worrisome picture of a high experience of erosion overall in the permanent teeth, although the proportion of young people with dentine involvement was only 2%, very similar to the data for 16–24-year-olds from the 1998 adult survey.

What are the implications for those providing dental services to adults in the UK?

The overall trends reported in the adult dental health survey of 1998 give reason for some optimism. However, closer inspection of the data reveals considerable shortcomings in the way in which oral and dental disease are managed in adults in the UK. Young adults have little evidence of dental intervention which is good, providing that is appropriate; what is disquieting is the way in which dental caries is mismanaged in the younger cohorts where 50% have untreated decay, visual or cavitated.

The inclusion of an assessment of 'visual' caries for the first time obviously raises issues about the usefulness or otherwise of doing so, given that surveys have a limited use for needs assessment and service utilisation and, inclusion of this assessment also increases the costs of surveys. In a number of populations 'visual' caries is going to be more prevalent, especially in young people,[10] but many of these lesions may remain static or regress; we do not know since this depends on conducting well-designed longitudinal studies. In terms of targeting populations for preventive measures, the balance between visual and cavitated lesions becomes important; if they are present in higher numbers than cavitated lesions, a sealant/preventive resin restoration programme is to be advocated. If, however, they are present in equal proportions then the implication is that caries progression is relatively rapid and a fluoride-based preventive programme would be more appropriate.

Fluorides and sealant based preventive programmes may make an impact in certain areas, but the role of hygiene in preventing dental caries should not be ignored either. This applies particularly to caries on free smooth surfaces, specifically perhaps to the emerging issue of root surface caries in older adults. Despite a multi-million pound oral hygiene industry and regular dental attendance amongst a majority of the adult population, evidence from elsewhere in this survey[6] suggests that there is still a widespread problem with hygiene. The reported frequency of toothbrushing had little effect on periodontal disease and, even amongst the majority of people who purported to be regular tooth-brushers, the prevalence of visible plaque deposits was still very high. The profession still has a key role to play here too.

The pattern of disease and the emphasis of treatment does seem to be changing. In younger adults there are fewer restorations than hitherto and simple, minimally damaging techniques may be appropriate to manage disease. In older adults there are more restorations, often large, complex and requiring time and advanced professional skills to maintain. The evidence that change is needed in the way treatment is delivered to reflect this is compelling. Innovations, such as the development of a greater role for PCDs, may offer some of the solutions for managing this changed environment.

This article has been refereed under the British Dental Journal reviewing process. Full details of sample numbers and the criteria for the clinical examinations can be found in the survey report. We would like to acknowledge the work of Alison Walker, Maureen Kelly and other staff of the Office for National Statistics. This work was undertaken by a consortium comprising the Office for National Statistics and the Dental Schools of the Universities of Birmingham, Dundee, Newcastle and Wales who received funding from the United Kingdom Health Departments; the views expressed in this publication are those of the authors and not necessarily those of the Health Departments nor of the other members of the consortium.

1. Winn D M, Brunelle J A, Selwitz R H, Kaste L M, Oldakowski R J, Kingman A, Brown L J. Coronal and root caries in the dentition of adults in the United States, 1988-1991. *J Dent Res* 1996; **75**(Spec Issue): 642-651.
2. Schuller A A, Holst D. Changes in the oral health of adults from Trondelag, Norway, 1973-1983-1994. *Community Dent Oral Epidemiol* 1998; **26**; 201-208.
3. Berset G P, Eriksen H M, Bjertness E, Hansen B F. Caries experience of 35-year-old Oslo residents and changes over a 20-year period. *Community Dent Health* 1996; **13**: 238-244.
4. Hugoson A, Koch G, Slotte C, Bergendal T, Thorstensson B, Thorstensson H. caries prevalence and distribution in 20-80-year-olds in Jonkoping, Sweden, in 1973, 1983, 1993. *Community Dent Oral Epidemiol* 2000; **28**: 90-96.
5. Kalsbeek H, Truin G-J, Poorterman J H G, van Rossum G M J M, van Rikom H M, Verrips G H W. Trends in periodontal status and oral hygiene habits in Dutch adults between 1983 and 1995. *Community Dent Oral Epidemiol* 2000; **28**: 112-118.
6. Kelly M et al. *Adult Dental Health Survey. Oral Health in the United Kingdom in 1998.* London: The Stationery Office, 2000.
7. Steele J G. *National Diet and Nutrition survey: people aged 65 years and over. Volume 2: Report of the oral health survey.* London: The Stationery Office, 1998
8. Steele J G, Walls A W G. Partial recording systems for the assessment of tooth wear in older adults. *Community Dent Oral Epidemiol* 2000; **28**: 18-25.
9. O'Brien M. *Children's dental health in the United Kingdom 1993.* London: Her Majesty's Stationery Office, 1994.
10. Bjarnason S, Kohler B, Ranggard L. Dental caries in a group of 15-16-year-olds from Goteborg. Part 1. *Swed Dent J* 1992; **16**: 143-149.

Dental restorations in adults in the UK in 1998 and implications for the future

C. M. Pine,[1] N. B. Pitts,[2] J. G. Steele,[3] J. N. Nunn,[4] and E. Treasure,[5]

People in their late fifties in the UK today can expect to live another 20 years and most want to maintain a functional and aesthetically acceptable dentition. However, 50% of the teeth of dentate adults aged 45 years and over are filled and crowned. The challenges for the dental profession in addressing these aspirations are discussed.

[1]*Reader in Dental Public Health, Head of Section of Dental Public Health & Health Psychology, University of Dundee;* [2]*Professor and Unit Director, Dental Health Services Research Unit, University of Dundee;* [3]*Senior Lecturer in Restorative Dentistry, University of Newcastle upon Tyne;* [4]*Senior Lecturer in Child Dental Health, University of Newcastle upon Tyne;* [5]*Professor of Dental Public Health, University of Wales*
Correspondence to : Cynthia Pine, Head of Section of Dental Public Health & Health Psychology, The Dental School, University of Dundee, Park Place, Dundee DD1 4HR
email: c.m.pine@dundee.ac.uk
REFEREED PAPER
Received 13.06.00; Accepted 31.07.00
© *British Dental Journal* 2001; **190:** 4–8

The national surveys of Adult Dental Health have given a 10-yearly summary of the clinical condition of adults in the United Kingdom on three previous occasions. The fourth report in the series was published in March of 2000. For the 1998 survey 4,984 addresses were identified at which all adults over 16 in residence were asked to take part in the survey; 21% of households refused and no contact was made at 5% of them. In total, 6,204 adults were interviewed following which those with some teeth were asked to undergo a dental examination; 3,817 (72%) of those eligible agreed. A weighting system based on some of the interview responses of those who consented to be dentally examined and those who were interviewed but not dentally examined was used to reduce bias from non-response.[13] The survey was carried out under the auspices of the Office of National Statistics together with the Universities of Birmingham, Dundee, Newcastle-upon-Tyne and Wales.

After being interviewed, adults with some natural teeth were asked whether they would consent to a dental examination in their own home. This paper presents and discusses the results of these examinations in terms of the numbers and distribution of filled teeth, artificial crowns and root surface restorations recorded. Each examiner was trained and calibrated in the diagnostic criteria prior to the survey. Examinations were conducted with adults seated and examiners using illumination from a dental overhead 'Daray' light. A mirror and ball-ended CPI probe were used, but teeth were not dried with compressed air and no radiographs were taken. For each filled or crowned tooth, the examiner was required to indicate the status of the restoration as filled and sound, filled with recurrent caries, or filled with a failed but not carious restoration. For the first time in the accompanying report to this survey,[1] crowns were reported separately to fillings. This paper considers each component of adults' dental restorations, ie fillings within the crown, artificial crowns and fillings in the root surfaces and reports the pattern of restorations amongst United Kingdom adults in 1998, as well as discussing how this pattern is likely to change in future generations and the implications of these changes for the dental profession.

In brief
- Almost one in three young adults (16–24 years) have no fillings
- Overall, 90% of all dentate adults in 1998 had at least one filling with people on average having seven filled teeth
- One third of dentate adults in the UK had at least one crown
- Over one third of those aged 55 and over had root surface fillings

Are fillings becoming a feature of middle age?

The decline in dental caries experience amongst children in the United Kingdom and western Europe over the past 20 years is well documented.[2] This improvement in child dental health can now be seen in the youngest adult cohort examined in the 1998 survey. Almost 1 in 3 young adults (31% aged 16 to 24 years) have no filled teeth. This is in stark contrast to the next cohort, aged 25 to 34, of whom only 4% have no fillings (Table 1).

Despite the good news in relation to young people, overall 90% of all dentate adults in 1998 had at least one filled tooth with people on average having seven filled teeth. Adults are living longer and keeping their teeth for longer. If we compare 1988 with 1998, the group with the biggest increase in the average number of teeth were people aged 55 and over. They have about two more teeth, from 16.9 in 1988 to 18.8 in 1998. These figures refer only to the dentate population. However, in addition to dentate people having more teeth, substantially more people have any teeth. Therefore, the scale of the increase in the total number of teeth in this population age group is even greater than these average numbers suggest. Since this generation of people had higher disease levels historically, many of the teeth that have been retained have already been filled. In fact, over a third of all the teeth of middle aged adults are filled teeth. Good maintenance and prevention of further disease will be aided if dentists continue to provide restorations of high quality to this age group, as people in their late fifties today have an average life expectancy of another 20 years.

Within England, people living in the least deprived areas have the highest number of

A guide to the UK adult dental health survey 1998

Table 1	Distribution and mean number of filled (otherwise sound) teeth by age

Dentate adults							United Kingdom
	Age						All
Number of filled (otherwise sound)	16–24	25–34	35–44	45–54	55–64	65 and over	
	%	%	%	%	%	%	%
None	31	4	3	3	9	14	10
1–5	53	38	22	17	31	34	32
6–11	15	45	48	48	39	37	40
12 or more	1	12	27	32	21	15	18
Mean number of filled (otherwise sound) teeth	2.6	6.6	8.8	9.3	7.4	6.3	7.0
Base	491	854	781	746	461	484	3817

restored teeth with an average of 8.6. These people were also the group who were most likely to want to keep their teeth for life. Inevitably, some of these fillings will need replacing in the future. Overall, secondary caries remains the most commonly cited reason for replacing fillings.[3,4] However, mechanical failure of both cusps and fillings in previously restored teeth is increasingly reported for middle aged and older adult patients attending dental practice. More practice-based research is indicated in older adults to clarify their likely pattern of restorative failure.

On the positive side, this group of adults are best placed and best motivated to respond to preventive dental care. All these factors suggest that the dental team should be supported and encouraged to place emphasis on prevention of new disease for middle aged and elderly adults, so reducing their potential for developing secondary coronal and root caries.

Who is most likely to have filled teeth?

Women attend the dentist more regularly than men and continue to have more fillings, an average of 7.3 compared with 6.6. Again, the largest difference in who has filled teeth, occurred for those aged between 45 and 64. People in these age groups who attended the dentist for check-ups, either on an occasional or regular basis, had significantly more teeth than those who only attended when they had a dental problem. The result of saving all these teeth has been that dentists have filled rather than extracted many of them, and people who attended for dental check-ups showed that benefit by ending up with most teeth and most fillings (Table 2).

There were differences around the country with higher disease levels in the north and west of the United Kingdom. The biggest contrast was seen in those aged 35 to 44 years. In England, 25% of these adults had 12 or more filled teeth compared with 49% in Northern Ireland (Table 3).

Filled teeth are still more common amongst adults from non-manual backgrounds, but the differences between the social groups has reduced over the past 20 years. People from non-manual backgrounds have reduced their average number of filled teeth from 9.9 in 1978 to 8.9 in 1998. In contrast, those from manual backgrounds have increased their average from 5.9 in 1978 to 6.6 in 1998. One of the contributing factors is likely to be the increase in the proportion of people attending for regular check-ups. In 1978, only 28% of those from unskilled manual backgrounds reported attending regularly compared with 49% in 1998. This change has been much less for those from non-manual backgrounds, from 56% in 1978 to 65% in 1998.

In summary, those who have most filled teeth are people aged 35 years and over, women, people from non-manual backgrounds, and those who reported regular dental attendance.

How likely are fillings to be sound and made of amalgam?

The condition of fillings is an important consideration, particularly amongst the

Table 2	Twelve or more filled (otherwise sound) teeth by usual reason for dental attendance and age

Dentate adults				United Kingdom
Age	Usual reason for attendance			
	Regular check-up	Occasional check-up	Only with trouble	All
	Percentage with 12 or more filled (otherwise sound) teeth			
16–24	0	2	2	1
25–34	15	12	8	12
35–44	31	31	14	27
45–54	38	23	18	32
55–64	29	–	4	21
65 and over	21	–	0	15
All	24	15	8	18

Dental restorations

Table 3	Twelve or more filled (otherwise sound) teeth by country and age				
Dentate adults					
Age	Country				United Kingdom
	England	Wales	Scotland	Northern Ireland	
	Percentage with 12 or more filled (otherwise sound) teeth				
16–24	0	3	4	8	1
25–34	10	10	26	26	12
35–44	25	32	34	49	27
45–54	32	31	29	37	32
55–64	21	18	21	20	21
65 and over	15	11	11	16	15
All	18	18	23	27	18
Base	2186	502	668	461	3817

middle-aged and elderly dentate people, who have successfully retained their teeth but at the cost of having them filled. During the survey dental examinations, teeth with fillings (or crowns) were classified as sound fillings, unsound fillings or filled with caries. An unsound filling or failed restoration was deemed failed not because of caries, if the restoration was chipped, cracked or had a margin into which a ball-ended probe tip would fit. In general, this meant that all major physical defects were included. The survey will have given an underestimation of teeth with recurrent caries as no radiographs were taken.

Encouragingly, only 4% of all fillings were judged to be mechanically unsound. On average, dentate adults had 7.6 teeth with fillings, 7.1 were judged sound, 0.3 unsound and 0.2 to have further decay. An added bonus was that older people's fillings were no more likely to be judged unsound than fillings in young people.

The overwhelming majority of filled teeth were restored with silver amalgam, 84% of all filled teeth. Of these, only 3% were judged unsound, again with little variation with age.

Whose teeth are most likely to be crowned?

One third of dentate adults in the United Kingdom had at least one crowned tooth (34%). Most people with crowns had one or two crowns (20%), but 5% had at least six.

People with most crowns were aged 45 to 54 years and nearly half of that age group had a crown (Fig. 1). Regular attenders in this age group also had an average of three more teeth compared with people who only attend the dentist when they have a problem. In fact, middle aged dentate adults (45 to 64) were nearly 15 times more likely to have a crown than young adults (< 25 years). The effects of a lifetime of dental care may well have contributed to the retention of teeth; albeit in this age group, that to keep these teeth more may have needed to be crowned.

Regular dental attenders had most crowns (40%) compared with those attending only when they have a problem (23%). More women than men had crowns, 37% compared with 31%. However, there were no regional differences and similar numbers of people around the UK had crowns. As might be expected, there were differences between social groups. People living in households headed by those in non-manual occupations were more likely to have crowns (38%) than those from unskilled occupations (28%). The number of people with crowns has increased markedly across all social groups since the 1988 survey, with the largest increase occurring in those from unskilled manual backgrounds.

How common are root surface fillings?

Overall, 15% of dentate adults had root surface filings in 1998. Clearly, the reasons for placement were not known and will be a combination of root surface caries and tooth wear. Inevitably, older people had more root surface fillings with none recorded in those under 25, an average of 0.5 teeth with fillings in those aged 45 to 54 and 1.3 for those aged 65 years and older.

The proportions of people with root surface fillings rose steadily with 35% of 55-64 year olds and 43% of those aged 65 and above (Table 4). The severity rose also, so that many more teeth were affected in the oldest age group with 6% having six or more teeth with root surface fillings. It is salutary to remember that in 1968, only 21% of people aged 65–74 had any teeth compared with

A guide to the UK adult dental health survey 1998

66% in 1998. Tooth retention with advancing years is leading to more complex dental restorative challenges for dentists caring for our aging population.

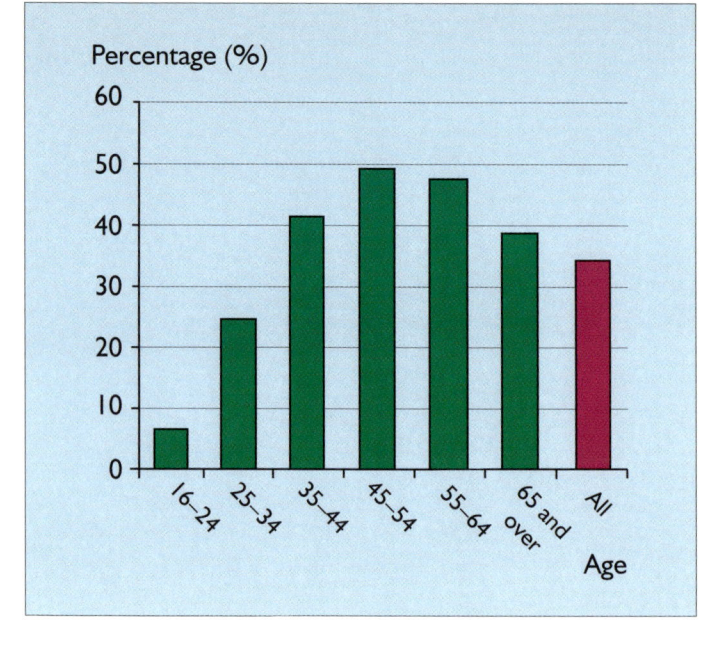

Fig. 1 Proportion of dentate adults with one or more artificial crowns by age

What are the implications for general dental practitioners in the near future?

To begin to address this question, it is helpful to have a complete picture of restorations in 1998. So far, this paper has considered fillings, crowns and root surface fillings separately. The total number of restorations in the crowns and root surfaces of teeth is given in Table 5 by age group.

Probably, the most useful statistic is the average proportion of restored teeth by age. For those aged 16 to 24 years, only 11% of their teeth are restored. Over the next 10 years, this cohort can be expected to maintain relatively better dental health than the previous generation as expectations and healthy habits continue to improve. Undoubtedly, the key age groups most impacting on dentists' working life will be adults in their middle years.

Other northern European countries are facing similar general and dental demographic profiles, ie an ageing, dentate population.[5] In 1999, Norwegian public health dentists examined future demand for dental care in Norway from a macro-economic perspective.[6] They predicted that there would be an increase in demand for dental services over the next 10–15 years, with an increasing proportion of elderly dentate people demanding more services. From 2010–15, they felt that picture would change as the younger age groups with fewer fillings get older. However, it should be noted that Scandinavian countries have much narrower differences in wealth (and health) between the richest and poorest people compared with the UK. Of concern, for our own aging UK population will be the continuation of a divide in the health of the elderly and in their economic power to pay for healthcare. In the UK, Richard Scase[7] has developed scenarios for 2010 from a social science perspective. His report predicted future over 50s acting younger with a core of 'time rich, cash rich' middle aged consumers. These groups are likely to want to maintain a functional and aesthetically acceptable dentition. However, there will continue to be a significant minority of older adults living in poverty, which may limit their ability to access care. This problem is faced and has been considered for some time in the United States. Those reviewing care of the dentate elderly have suggested that linking dental primary care services with other primary health services like hearing and vision may support future national funding priorities.[8] This would put the maintenance and restoration of oral function into an overall context of improving quality of life.

A further note of caution is needed as for some people, longevity will be at the cost of multiple drug regimes or polypharmacy. In

Table 4	Distribution and mean number of teeth with root surface fillings by age						
Dentate adults							United Kingdom
Number of teeth with root surface fillings	Age						
	16–24	25–34	35–44	45–54	55–64	65 and over	All
	%	%	%	%	%	%	%
None	100	96	92	80	65	57	85
1–5	0	4	7	18	32	37	14
6–11	0	0	1	1	3	5	2
12 or more	0	0	0	0	0	1	0
Mean	0	0.1	0.2	0.5	0.9	1.3	0.4
Base	491	854	781	746	461	484	3817

Dental restorations

Table 5 Distribution and mean number of all teeth with any coronal or root restorations

Dentate adults *United Kingdom*

Number of teeth with any coronal or root restorations	Age						
	16–24	25–34	35–44	45–54	55–64	65 and over	All
	%	%	%	%	%	%	%
None	29	4	2	2	6	7	8
1–5	52	28	14	10	20	30	25
6–11	18	46	40	33	32	30	34
12 or more	2	22	44	56	43	32	33
Mean number of restored teeth	3.1	7.9	10.7	12.0	9.9	8.6	8.8
Mean number of teeth	27.9	28.1	26.7	24.0	19.9	17.3	24.8
Mean proportion of restored teeth	11	28	40	50	50	49	35
Base	491	854	781	746	461	484	3817

1976, 309 million prescriptions were dispensed compared with 505 million in 1997. Polypharmacy may result in reduced salivary flow and increasing vulnerability to root caries.[9] Although more people will retain vigour and good health with age, others will lose their ability for self care as they reach their seventies and eighties but, will still be dentate. The carers of these frail, elderly, dentate adults will need to be shown how to maintain oral hygiene.

In summary, in 1998, 50% of middle aged adults in the UK had teeth with fillings and many will keep these teeth for life. Maintaining these adults' dentitions in good health will continue to be a challenge. This work will require expert technical care to replace failed restorations and the provision of appropriate preventive advice for patients to keep the need for new restorations to a minimum, especially root surface restorations. These twin challenges require different skills and dental practitioners should consider how best both aspects can be delivered within their practice.

Prevention of new root carious lesions will require careful advice on oral hygiene maintenance and a healthy diet.[10] Investing in prevention for middle aged and older adults is a new area for dentists and for those funding dental services. Commissioners of dental care will need to recognise that initial costs of prevention may well be greater than treatment costs but investing in maintaining health will not only help older adults to keep their teeth for as long as possible, but will also have a major impact on maintenance costs. There is clearly potential for dental hygienists, therapists and dental health educators to play a part within these more challenging treatment plans.

This article has been refereed under the British Dental Journal reviewing process. Full details of sample numbers and the criteria for the clinical examinations can be found in the survey report. We would like to acknowledge the work of Alison Walker, Maureen Kelly and other staff of the Office for National Statistics. This work was undertaken by a consortium comprising the Office for National Statistics and the Dental Schools of the Universities of Birmingham, Dundee, Newcastle and Wales who received funding from the United Kingdom Health Departments; the views expressed in this publication are those of the authors and not necessarily those of the Health Departments nor of the other members of the consortium.

1. Kelly M, Steele J, Bradnock G et al. Adult Dental Health. *Oral Health in the United Kingdom 1998*. London: The Stationery Office, 2000.
2. Pine C M. *Community Oral Health*. Oxford: Butterworth-Heinemann. 1997.
3. Pink F E, Minden N J, Simmonds S. Decisions of practitioners regarding placement of amalgam and composite restorations in general practice settings. *Oper Dent* 1994; **19** : 127-132.
4. Burke F J, Cheung S W, Mjor I A, Wilson N H. Restoration longevity and analysis of reasons for the palcement and replacement of restorations provided by vocational dental practitioners and their trainers in the United Kingdom. *Quintessence Int* 1999; **30**: 234-242.
5. Kalsbeek H, Truin G J van Rossum G M, van Rijkom H M, Pooterman J H, Verrips G H. Trends in caries prevalence in Dutch adults between 1983 and 1995. *Caries Res* 1998; **32**: 160-165.
6. Grytten J, Lund E. Future demand for dental care in Norway; a macro-economic perspective. *Comm Dent Oral Epidemiol* 1999; **27**: 321-330.
7. Scase R. *Britain towards 2010. A report of the Foresight Programme Leisure and Learning Panel of the Economic and Social Science Research Council*. London: ESRC, 1999.
8. Jones J A, Adelson R, Niessen L C, Gilbert G H. Issues in financing dental care for the elderly. *J Public Health Dent* 1990; **50**: 268-275.
9. Jones J A. Root caries: prevention and chemotherapy. *Am J Dent* 1995; **8**: 352-357.
10. Fedele D J, Sheets C G. Issues in the treatment of root caries in older adults. *J Esthet Dent* 1998; **10**: 243-252.

Factors associated with oral health: a multivariate analysis of results from the 1998 Adult Dental Health survey

E. Treasure,[1] M. Kelly,[2] N. Nuttall,[3] J. Nunn,[4] G. Bradnock,[5] and D. White[6]

This paper presents results from the 1998 Adult Dental Health Survey using multivariate analysis. This enables analysis of several variables at one time to see which are having an effect on people's oral health. The paper compares these variables to a variety of outcome measures and makes recommendations for dental practice.

The national surveys of Adult Dental Health have given a 10-yearly summary of the clinical condition of adults in the United Kingdom on three previous occasions. The fourth report in the series was published in March of 2000. For the 1998 survey 4,984 addresses were identified at which all adults over 16 in residence were asked to take part in the survey; 21% of households refused and no contact was made at 5% of them. In total, 6,204 adults were interviewed following which those with some teeth were asked to undergo a dental examination; 3,817 (72%) of those eligible agreed. A weighting system based on some of the interview responses of those who consented to be dentally examined and those who were interviewed but not dentally examined was used to reduce bias from non-response.[1] The survey was carried out under the auspices of the Office of National Statistics together with the Universities of Birmingham, Dundee, Newcastle-upon-Tyne and Wales.

The national surveys of adult dental health have tended to look at factors associated with oral health as single factors. For example the level of total tooth loss has been shown to be related to social class and to the part of the country people live in; but this raises the issue of whether differences in

In brief
- Variations in disease are caused by more than social class structure. It is likely that other complex socio-behavioural factors are at work.
- The survey supports the use of fissure sealants and encouraging people to brush their teeth more frequently.
- There is a huge difference in the experience of restorative dentistry in the average 20-year-old compared with the average 30-year-old.

total tooth loss patterns between countries is simply because they have different social class structures. In statistics there are a group of tests (multivariate models) designed specifically to select out which socio-demographic or behavioural factors were associated with clinically measured aspects of oral health. The data on the clinical measures of oral health were analysed using age standardisation and two multivariate modelling techniques; multiple regression for continuous dependent variables (eg number of teeth) and logistic regression for dependent variables with two outcomes (eg had artificial crowns or did not have artificial crowns).

The factors used in the modelling were:

Socio-Demographic:
- Age
- Gender
- Social class of head of household
- Educational attainment
- English region (North, South, Midlands) and country (Scotland, Northern Ireland Wales)
- Marital status
- Economic status.

Behavioural
- Usual reason for dental attendance
- Frequency of tooth cleaning
- Use of additional methods for cleaning teeth (eg floss).

In the figures 'triangles' are used to indicate where a variable was entered into the model but found to have no effect. In the analysis used these variables were then dropped.

What characteristics are associated with total tooth loss?
Table 1 shows the likelihood of a person with a given characteristic (eg a person from Scotland) having no natural teeth. The 'odds ratio' is simply the number of times more likely it is that a particular type of person will have no teeth in comparison to another. The 'another' person in this table is the one whose odds are 1.00. For example, for people of different ages those aged over 75 were 144 times more likely to have lost all their teeth in comparison with 16–44 year olds. Once all other factors in the model were taken into account educational attainment had the next largest effect after age on the odds of being edentate. The odds of being edentate were almost nine times higher for those adults with no qualification and four times higher for those with qualifications below degree level. Being from the north of Great Britain was also a factor that had an effect with the odds of having no teeth rising as distance from the South of England increased. The effect was not however observable in Northern Ireland. Gender was not found to be a factor that altered the odds of a person being edentate and this differs from the bivariate analysis.

What characteristics were associated with the number of natural teeth in the mouth?
Multiple regression modelling was carried out to discover which combinations of

---
[1]*Professor, University of Wales, Cardiff;* [2]*Senior Social Survey Officer, Office for National Statistics, London;* [3]*Senior Research Fellow, Dental Health Services Research Unit, University of Dundee;* [4]*Senior Lecturer, University of Newcastle upon Tyne;* [5]*Senior Lecturer,* [6]*Lecturer, University of Birmingham*
Correspondence to: Professor E T Treasure, The Dental School, Heath Park, Cardiff CF14 4XY email: treasureet@cardiff.ac.uk
REFEREED PAPER
Received 13.06.00; Accepted 31.07.00
© *British Dental Journal* 2001; **190:** 60–68

A guide to the UK adult dental health survey 1998

socio-demographic and behavioural factors independently affected the number of teeth among dentate adults (Fig. 1). The coefficients can be used to estimate the average number of teeth a person with given characteristics would have by adding them up for a person and adding this to a constant calculated by the model. For example, a 32-year-old married women who has a university degree and comes from a non-manual working background living in Scotland and who brushes her teeth twice a day and claims to attend for regular check-ups would be expected to have 28.44 teeth.

Constant	22.40
Age 25–34	+3.79
Woman	+0
Scotland	-0.85
Non-manual working background	+0.64
Degree	+0.99
Married	+0.40
Tooth cleaning twice daily	+0.54
Regular check-ups	+0.54
Total	28.44

Whether a person used an additional method of tooth cleaning was entered into the model but was not found to have any independent effect on the number of teeth among dentate adults.

It is often pointed out that the dental diseases are a largely preventable. So why, if this is the case, are people who live in Scotland likely to have 1.82 fewer teeth than someone from the South of England once all other factors are taken into account? Is there a factor simply in being from Scotland that could account for an almost two tooth disadvantage over the South of England? The answer is that other factors will be at work as well, which is indicated by the R^2 value that shows how much of the variation is explained by the model, in this case 44%. There are some obvious candidates that might add to the explanatory power of these models one of which would be dietary factors such as eating sugary foods or drinks.

What can this sort of analysis tell us about the experience of dental disease among young adults?

Adults under the age of 35 were found to have a relatively low experience of dental disease and treatment. By concentrating on this group it was planned to exclude the historical burden of disease and concentrate on the factors associated with the number of sound and untreated teeth.

This analysis again indicated that age was the most important factor followed by region or country. However in the case of young adults it was the Midlands where people had most sound and untreated teeth on average and Northern Ireland where people had fewest. A potentially important finding was that those adults who had some fissure sealants had 1.32 more sound and untreated teeth than those who did not have sealants. This suggests that, at a population level, sealants play an effective role in preventing disease at this age. Only 24 % of the variation was explained by the factors included in this model (Fig. 2).

What factors are associated with having dental caries or unsound teeth?

Because of the huge proportion of subjects with no decayed or unsound teeth and that the remaining subjects had very few decayed teeth this oral health measure was treated as a dichotomous variable. This measure showed very different associations in comparison with the other clinical measurements. Firstly, there was a different relationship with age. People aged 25 to 34 and those aged 45 to 54 years were the only ones to have significantly greater odds of having a decayed or unsound tooth. Living in the north of Great Britain was again associated with poorer dental health: those in the north of England were 1.86 times more likely to have some untreated decay than those living in the south of England. Only one of the behavioural variables varied significantly between groups and that was,

Table 1 Likelihood of an adult having lost all their natural teeth (based on odds ratios from logistic regression)

Dentate adults — United Kingdom

Characteristic	Odds ratio
16–44	1.00
45–54	10.77‡
55–64	34.05‡
65–74	71.95‡
75 and over	144.05‡
English region or country	
North	2.02‡
Midlands	1.59‡
South	1.00
Wales	1.92†
Scotland	3.46‡
Northern Ireland	1.47
Social class of head of household	
I, II, IIINM	1.00
IIIM	2.14‡
IV, V	2.21‡
Educational attainment	
At degree level or above	1.00
Below degree level	3.95‡
No qualifications	8.79‡
Marital status	
Single	1.45*
Married/cohabiting	1.00
Divorced/separated	1.43
Widowed	1.62‡
R^2	0.50

*Significant at 95% level
†Significant at 99% level
‡Significant at 99.9% level

Factors associated with oral health

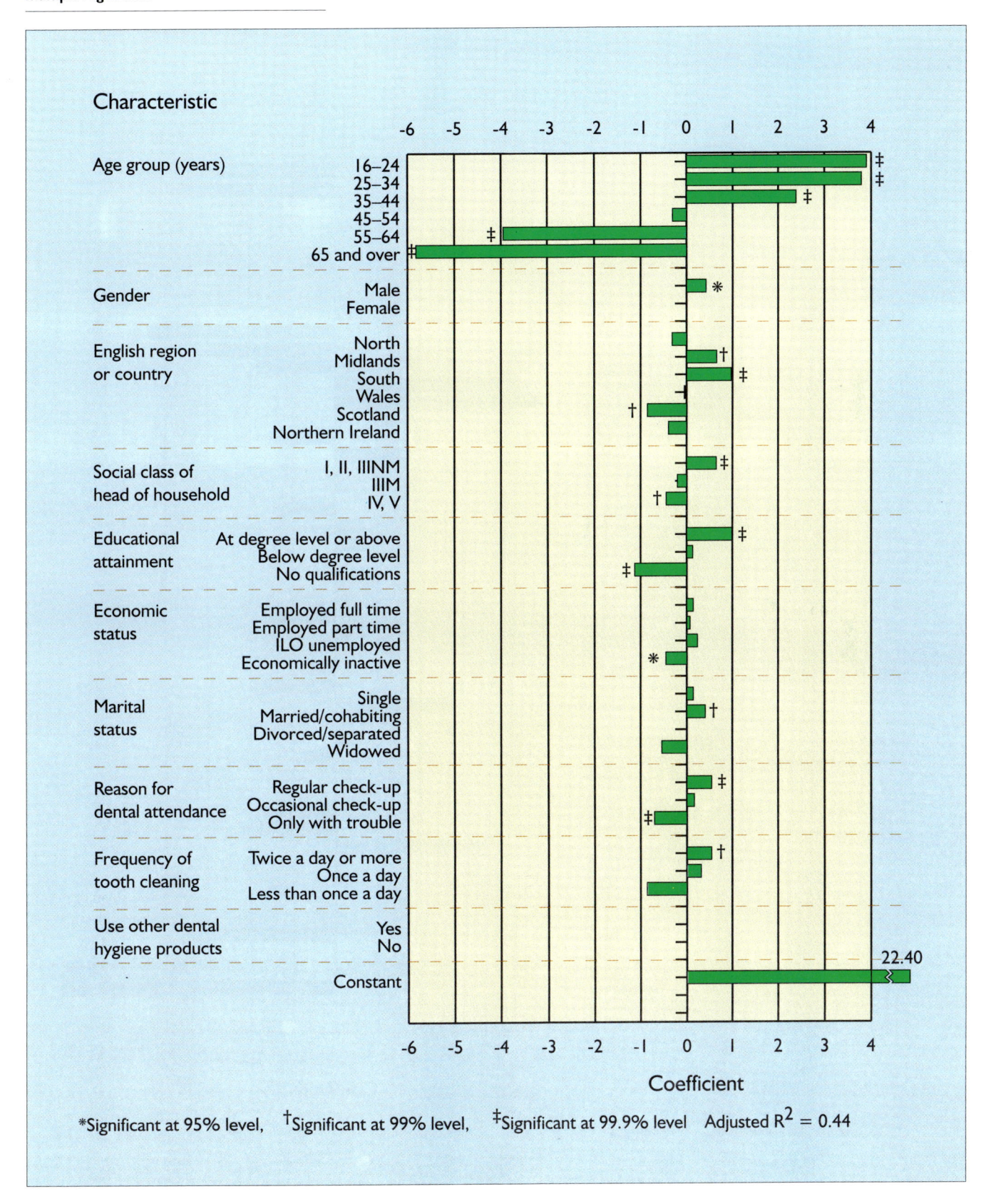

Fig. 1 Factors independently affecting the number of teeth based on coefficients from multiple regression

Characteristic		Coefficient	Significance
Age group (years)	16–24	~3.9	‡
	25–34	~3.8	‡
	35–44	~2.7	‡
	45–54	~-0.3	
	55–64	~-3.7	‡
	65 and over	~-6.2	‡
Gender	Male	~0.4	*
	Female		
English region or country	North	~-0.1	
	Midlands	~0.8	†
	South	~1.2	‡
	Wales	~0	
	Scotland	~-1.0	†
	Northern Ireland	~-0.3	
Social class of head of household	I, II, IIINM	~1.0	‡
	IIIM	~0.1	
	IV, V	~-0.5	†
Educational attainment	At degree level or above	~1.5	‡
	Below degree level	~0.2	
	No qualifications	~-1.5	‡
Economic status	Employed full time	~0.1	
	Employed part time	~-0.2	
	ILO unemployed	~0.3	
	Economically inactive	~-0.6	*
Marital status	Single	~0.2	
	Married/cohabiting	~0.7	†
	Divorced/separated	~-0.4	
	Widowed	~-0.3	
Reason for dental attendance	Regular check-up	~1.0	‡
	Occasional check-up	~0.2	
	Only with trouble	~-1.1	‡
Frequency of tooth cleaning	Twice a day or more	~0.7	†
	Once a day	~0.3	
	Less than once a day	~-0.9	
Use other dental hygiene products	Yes	~0.3	
	No		
Constant		22.40	

*Significant at 95% level, †Significant at 99% level, ‡Significant at 99.9% level   Adjusted R^2 = 0.44

A guide to the UK adult dental health survey 1998

Fig. 2 Factors independently affecting the numbers of sound and untreated teeth (based on coefficients from multiple regression)

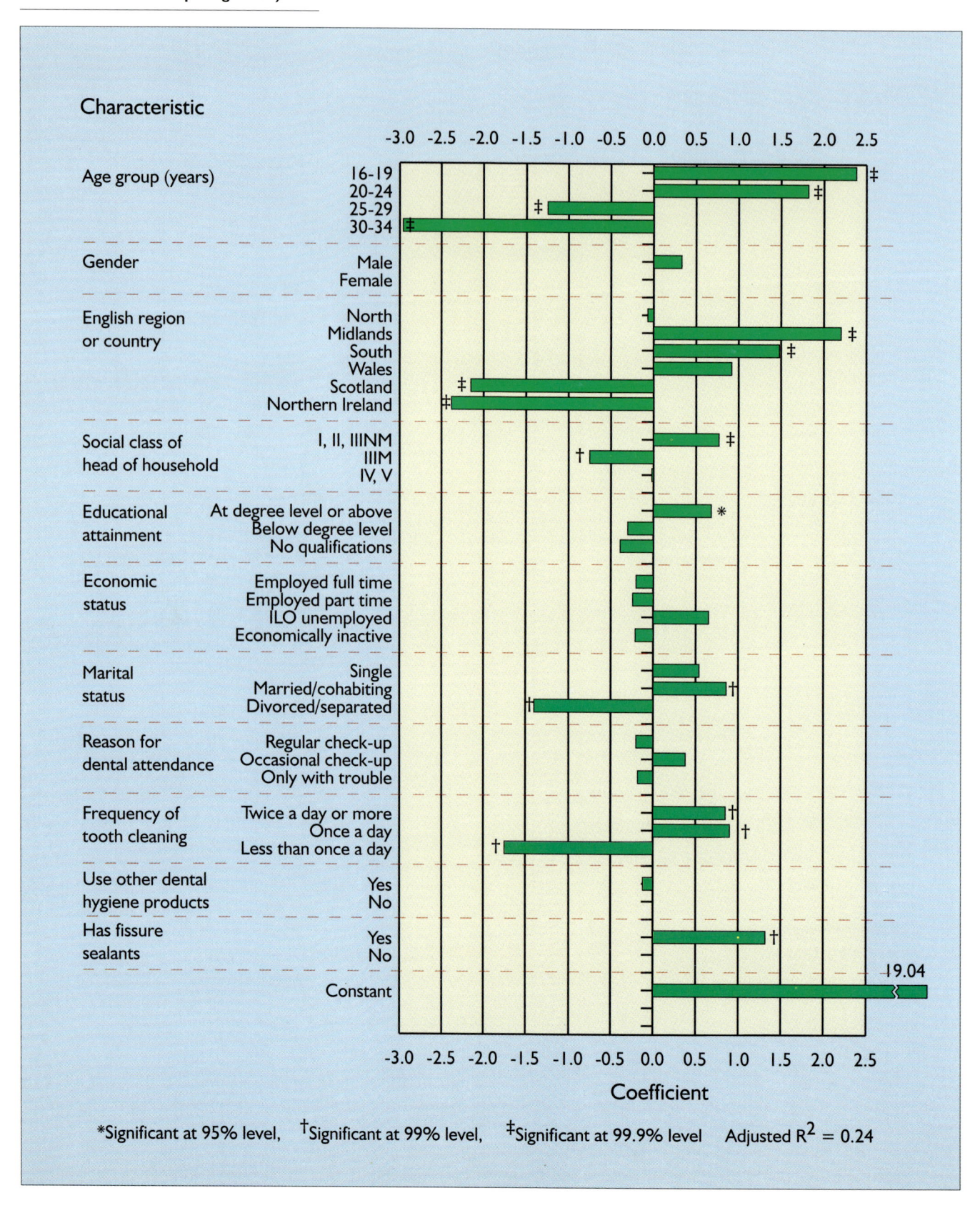

Characteristic		Coefficient
Age group (years)	16-19	2.4 ‡
	20-24	1.8 ‡
	25-29	-1.3 ‡
	30-34	-2.9 ‡
Gender	Male	—
	Female	0.2
English region or country	North	-0.1
	Midlands	2.1 ‡
	South	1.6 ‡
	Wales	0.8
	Scotland	-1.8 ‡
	Northern Ireland	-2.6 ‡
Social class of head of household	I, II, IIINM	0.8 ‡
	IIIM	0.4 †
	IV, V	—
Educational attainment	At degree level or above	0.9 *
	Below degree level	-0.2
	No qualifications	-0.3
Economic status	Employed full time	-0.1
	Employed part time	-0.2
	ILO unemployed	0.5
	Economically inactive	0.1
Marital status	Single	0.4
	Married/cohabiting	0.9 †
	Divorced/separated	-1.2
Reason for dental attendance	Regular check-up	-0.1
	Occasional check-up	0.3
	Only with trouble	—
Frequency of tooth cleaning	Twice a day or more	0.9 †
	Once a day	0.9 †
	Less than once a day	-1.0 †
Use other dental hygiene products	Yes	-0.1
	No	—
Has fissure sealants	Yes	1.3 †
	No	—
Constant		19.04

*Significant at 95% level, †Significant at 99% level, ‡Significant at 99.9% level   Adjusted $R^2 = 0.24$

Factors associated with oral health

Fig. 3 Likelihood of an adult having decayed and unsound teeth or unrestorable teeth (based on odds ratio from logistic regression)

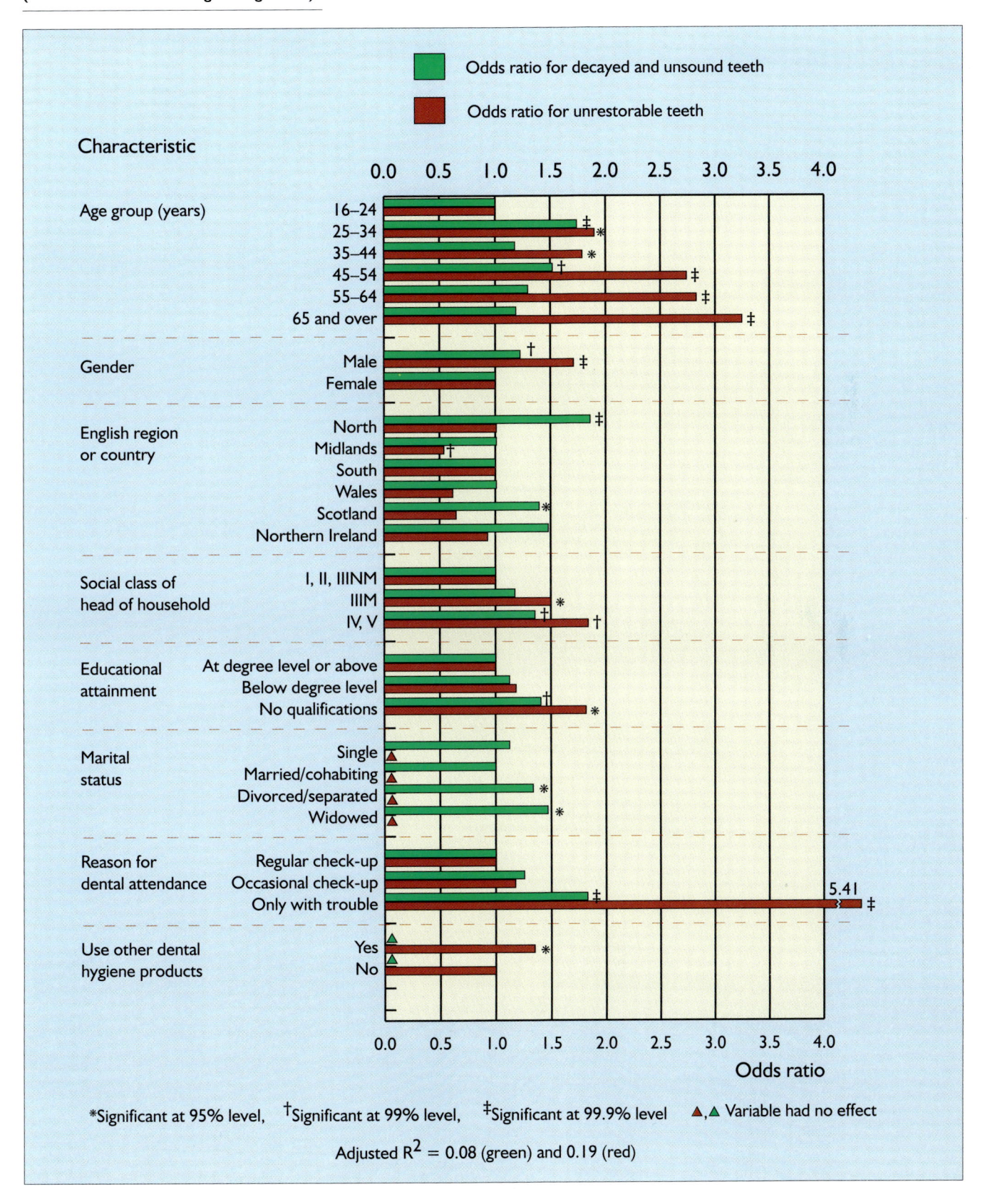

- Odds ratio for decayed and unsound teeth
- Odds ratio for unrestorable teeth

Characteristic	
Age group (years)	16–24, 25–34, 35–44, 45–54, 55–64, 65 and over
Gender	Male, Female
English region or country	North, Midlands, South, Wales, Scotland, Northern Ireland
Social class of head of household	I, II, IIINM; IIIM; IV, V
Educational attainment	At degree level or above, Below degree level, No qualifications
Marital status	Single, Married/cohabiting, Divorced/separated, Widowed
Reason for dental attendance	Regular check-up, Occasional check-up, Only with trouble (5.41)
Use other dental hygiene products	Yes, No

*Significant at 95% level, †Significant at 99% level, ‡Significant at 99.9% level, ▲,▲ Variable had no effect

Adjusted R^2 = 0.08 (green) and 0.19 (red)

A guide to the UK adult dental health survey 1998

Fig. 4 Likelihood of a dentate adult having 12 or more restored (otherwise sound) teeth or having artificial crowns (based on odds ratios from logistic regression)

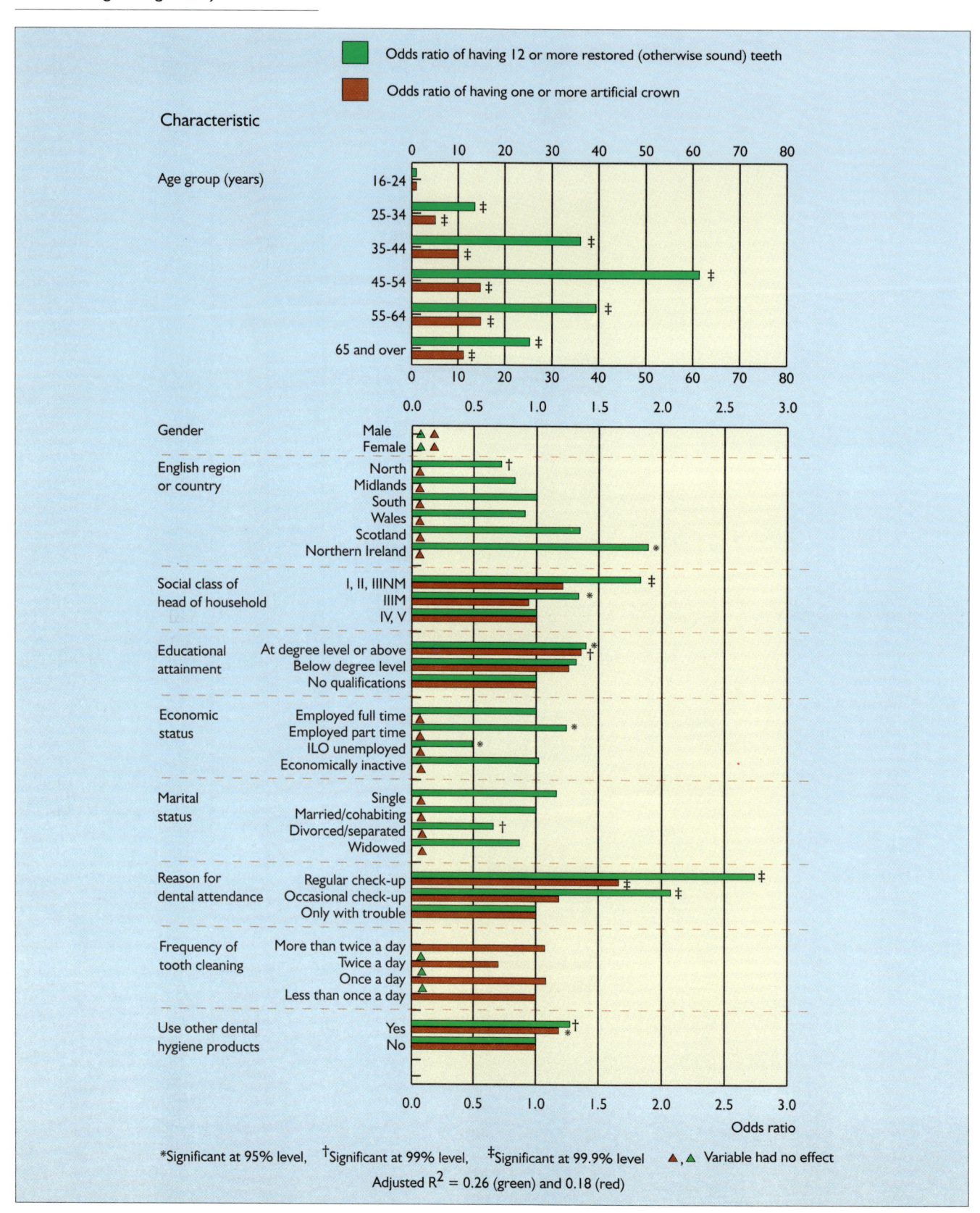

those who reported attending the dentist only with trouble had significantly higher odds of having a decayed or unsound tooth. Factors that were not found to be significant by the model were whether people were in employment or not, frequency of tooth cleaning and the use of additional dental hygiene products along with toothbrush or toothpaste. It is clear that as only 8% of the model was explained there are many factors influencing this measure that are not included in this analysis (Fig. 3).

The picture for unrestorable decay was different. The factor that had the strongest association with having unrestorable caries was the reported attendance pattern at a dentist. People who said they attended only when they had trouble had odds five times higher than those who said they went to the dentist for a regular check-up. The other strong relationship was with age where the odds increased with age so that at age 65 the odds were over 3 times greater than at age 16 to 24. People in the Midlands had significantly lower odds of having an unrestorable tooth in comparison with the other regions and countries of the United Kingdom. Women were also less likely to have some unrestorable caries in comparison with men. Marital status, economic status or reported frequency of tooth cleaning were not significant factors. The model explained 19% of the variation.

What factors are associated with the experience of restorative treatment in adults?

Two measures were used to try to gain some understanding of the factors underlying adults who have had some restorative treatment. These were whether a person had 12 restored but otherwise sound teeth or if they had an artificial crown (Fig. 4).

As might be expected age was the most important factor in determining the odds of an adult having either 12 or more restored teeth or an artificial crown.

The chance of having 12 or more filled teeth increased markedly with age until 55; and then dropped. A dentate person aged 50 was over 60 times more likely to have 12 or more filled teeth than someone aged 20. However, more remarkable was the huge difference just between the two youngest age groups; the average 30-year-old was 13 times more likely to have 12 or more filled teeth than the average adult aged 20. This was a much more marked difference than between any other two consecutive age groups; 40-year-olds were only about 3 times more likely to have 12 or more filled teeth than 30-year-olds. This illustrates something that comes out in other analyses in the survey report which is that a new generation is entering the adult population who have much less experience of restorative treatment.

It should come as no surprise that dental attendance behaviour was a strong factor in the experience of having restorative treatment. Those adults who said they usually went to a dentist for regular check-ups were 2.74 times more likely to have 12 or more sound and restored teeth and 1.66 times more likely to have an artificial crown than those who said they only went to a dentist when having some dental trouble.

What factors are associated with periodontal conditions?

In the logistical regression for periodontal condition the measure used was loss of attachment of 4 mm or more (Fig. 5). Age was the factor most strongly related to periodontal conditions; adults over 65-years-old were 33 times more likely to have a loss of attachment of 4 mm or more in comparison with those aged 16 to 24. Men had significantly higher odds of having this degree of loss of attachment as did those with education below degree level. It is interesting that none of the behavioural factors that were examined were found to be significant in this model. Twenty-eight per cent of the variation is explained by this model.

Implications for the practice

This multivariate analysis gives some indication of the factors that may be responsible for variations in oral health. Living in Scotland or the north of England increases your chance of having lost all your teeth, or if you have some teeth, having some with dental caries. Furthermore, this association is not only caused by social class structure of the regions and countries of the United Kingdom which suggests that other more complex socio-behavioural factors are at work. Thus in order to bring about improvements in this area it is necessary to understand what these are. Findings such as these have also been described in other areas of healthcare.[2]

Trying to understand the reasons behind this variation can only be supposition in many instances but there are some interesting variations that may be worth looking at. For example why is Northern Ireland not a region associated with high levels of edentulousness or in having low numbers of teeth but does have significantly fewer sound and untreated teeth? Does this suggest a very different pattern of extraction in Northern Ireland more similar to the South of England although in other ways the disease pattern would appear to be very different from the south?

There are some tantalising suggestions in these data which it is not possible to substantiate. For example, is it only coincidence that the Midlands have the second highest coefficient for number of teeth and the greatest coefficient for the numbers of sound and untreated teeth? However this improved situation does not carry through to current decay or in the number of restorations. It is tempting to suggest that fluoride might be responsible for the greater chances of having more teeth and more healthy teeth but why not the other factors? It is not possible to say but it gives pointers for further research.

Why is there not an age relationship in the younger groups for unsound and untreated teeth? This suggests that the odds of having a decayed tooth are similar in these younger age groups. Does this mean that there is a problem accessing services or that as fast as these teeth are treated fresh decay is arising?

The findings regarding the effect of going to the dentist are quite difficult to interpret. Those who say they visit a dentist for regular check-ups have greater odds of having less decayed teeth, less unrestorable teeth but more filled teeth, more chance of having a crown and less sound and untreated teeth. It is all too easy to decide that these factors are caused by over-treatment but it is just not possible to deduce that from these data. This is because nothing is known about the

A guide to the UK adult dental health survey 1998

Fig. 5 Likelihood of a dentate adult having periodontal loss of attachment of 4 mm or more (based on odds ratio from logistic regression)

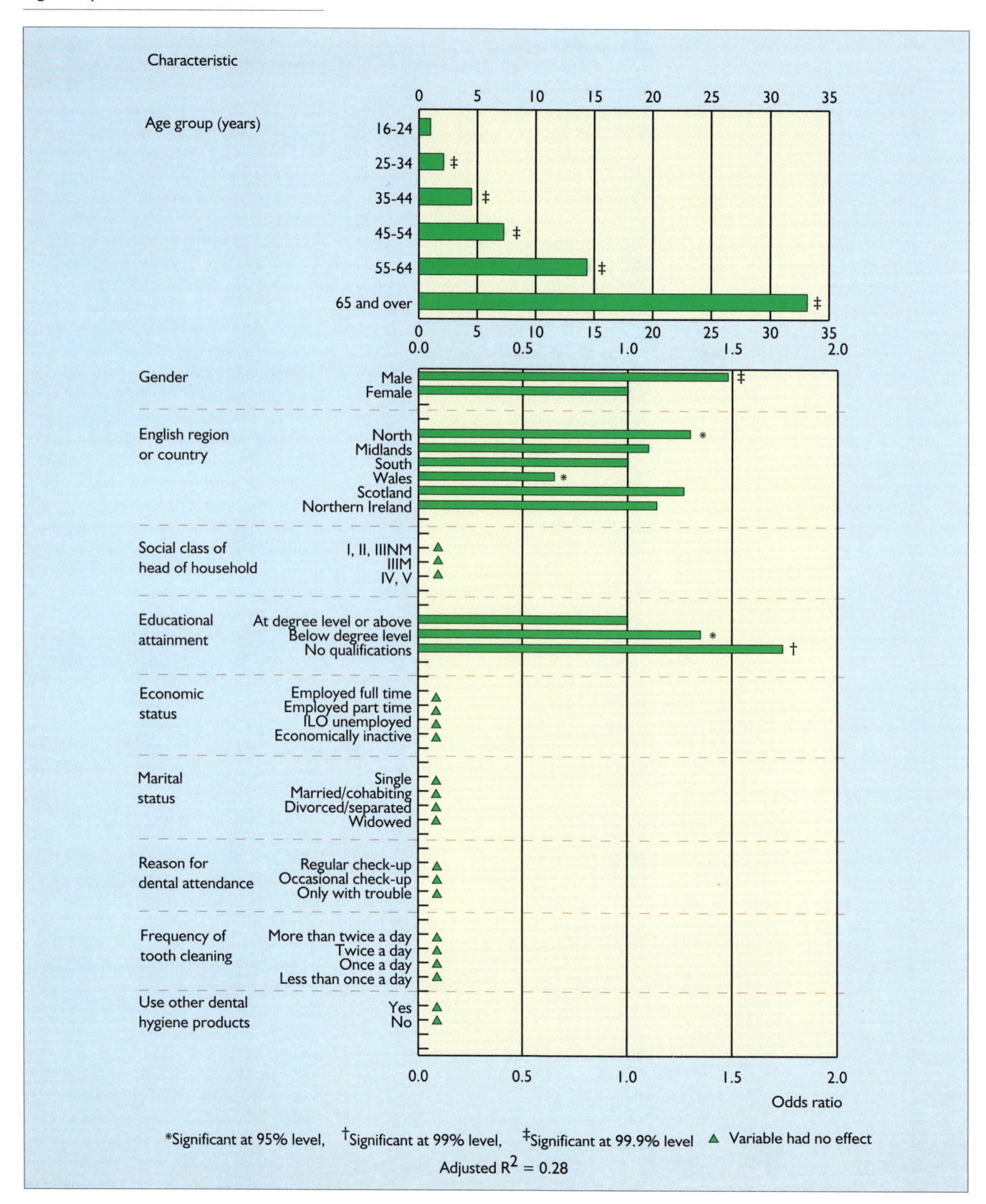

Characteristic		Odds ratio
Age group (years)	16-24	~1
	25-34	~2 ‡
	35-44	~4 ‡
	45-54	~7 ‡
	55-64	~15 ‡
	65 and over	~33 ‡
Gender	Male	‡
	Female	
English region or country	North	*
	Midlands	
	South	
	Wales	*
	Scotland	
	Northern Ireland	
Social class of head of household	I, II, IIINM	▲
	IIIM	▲
	IV, V	▲
Educational attainment	At degree level or above	
	Below degree level	*
	No qualifications	†
Economic status	Employed full time	▲
	Employed part time	▲
	ILO unemployed	▲
	Economically inactive	▲
Marital status	Single	▲
	Married/cohabiting	▲
	Divorced/separated	▲
	Widowed	▲
Reason for dental attendance	Regular check-up	▲
	Occasional check-up	▲
	Only with trouble	▲
Frequency of tooth cleaning	More than twice a day	▲
	Twice a day	▲
	Once a day	▲
	Less than once a day	▲
Use other dental hygiene products	Yes	▲
	No	▲

*Significant at 95% level, †Significant at 99% level, ‡Significant at 99.9% level, ▲ Variable had no effect

Adjusted $R^2 = 0.28$

incidence (as opposed to prevalence) of dental disease in this population and its subgroups. What has not been investigated here is the odds of having a functioning dentition related to reported attendance pattern. This is worthy of further investigation.

The findings relating to fissure sealants may be important in that they suggest that people who have fissure sealants in place are likely to have more sound and untreated teeth than others. However it is not possible to comment on the overall effectiveness of fissure sealing teeth as we do not know which other subjects had received sealants and then lost them or who had them replaced with a restoration. Similarly toothbrushing was positively associated with the number of sound and unrestored teeth.

Periodontal loss of attachment was not affected by any of the behavioural factors included in the models. It is unfortunate that smoking was omitted from the questionnaire and so could not be included. This does cause problems in how we should explain this disease to patients as there are no behavioural factors described here that can be recommended as making a real difference.

Being older was not associated with having a greater risk of having a decayed tooth but the oldest groups in this study did have a greater risk of having an unrestorable tooth. With the increasing proportion of the population who are ageing this must be of concern to the practitioner. What is to be done to reduce this more complex treatment need in the very oldest in society? Taken together it could be suggested that there is a need for a greater emphasis for a more preventive approach to dental practice. In particular the survey supports the use of fissure sealants and encouraging people to brush their teeth more frequently.

This article has been refereed under the British Dental Journal reviewing process. Full details of sample numbers and the criteria for the clinical examinations can be found in the survey report. We would like to acknowledge the work of Alison Walker and other staff of the Office for National Statistics.
This work was undertaken by a consortium comprising the Office for National Statistics and the Dental Schools of the Universities of Birmingham, Dundee, Newcastle and Wales who received funding from the United Kingdom Health Departments; the views expressed in this publication are those of the authors and not necessarily those of the Health Departments nor of the other members of the consortium.

1 Kelly M, Steele J, Nuttall N, Bradnock G, Morris J, Nunn J, Pine C, Pitts N, Treasure E, White D. *Adult Dental Health Survey — Oral Health in the United Kingdom 1998.* London: The Stationery Office, 2000.
2 Acheson D. *Independent Inquiry into Inequalities in Health.* The Stationery Office, ISBN 0 11 322173 8, 1998.

The impact of oral health on people in the UK in 1998

N. M. Nuttall,[1] J. G. Steele,[2] C. M. Pine,[3] D. White,[4] and N. B. Pitts[5]

Knowledge of the extent of dental disease gives a clinical indication of the experience of dental problems but it does not necessarily reflect the problems that people experience as a result of their dentition. It is becoming increasingly appreciated that the way a disease affects people's lives is just as important as epidemiological measures of its prevalence or incidence. The 1998 Adult Dental Health survey is the first of the decennial series of UK adult dental health surveys to use and report a measure of the self-perceived impact on people of the dental and periodontal diseases and other oral conditions. Over half (51%) of dentate adults said they had been affected in some way by their oral health, and in 8% of cases the impact was sufficient to have reduced their quality of life.

In brief
- Over half (51%) of dentate adults reported that an oral problem of some sort had affected them occasionally or more frequently in the 12 months preceding the survey.
- The most frequently experienced problem among dentate adults during the 12 months preceding the survey was oral pain (40%).
- The next most frequently experienced problems stemming from oral condition were psychological in nature (self-consciousness, feeling tense, difficulty relaxing or embarrassment)
- Eight per cent of dentate adults reported being severely affected by their oral health in that they felt their life was less satisfying or that they were totally unable to function at some time in the preceding year as a result of their oral condition.
- Many who had said they had experienced an oral problem in the preceding year had not gone to a dentist for treatment.

The national surveys of Adult Dental Health have given a 10-yearly summary of the clinical condition of adults in the United Kingdom on three previous occasions. The fourth report in the series was published in March of 2000. For the 1998 survey 4,984 addresses were identified at which all adults over 16 in residence were asked to take part in the survey; 21% of households refused and no contact was made at 5% of them. In total, 6,204 adults were interviewed following which those with some teeth were asked to undergo a dental examination: 3,817 (72%) of those eligible agreed. A weighting system based on some of the interview responses of those who consented to be dentally examined and those who were interviewed but not dentally examined was used to reduce bias from non-response.[1] The survey was carried out under the auspices of the Office of National Statistics together with the Universities of Birmingham, Dundee, Newcastle-upon-Tyne and Wales.

Preceding articles in this series have considered the clinical condition of teeth and supporting structures. However, clinical condition alone does not fully indicate how people feel affected by their oral state. In response to this a system to measure the impact of oral condition was introduced into the survey in 1998. This article considers some of these findings.

The oral health impact profile
The Oral Health Impact Profile (OHIP) scale is one of the dental family of health 'quality of life' scales that span the whole range of medical conditions.[2] These try to put some sort of numerical value on different health states or outcomes. OHIP is based on a model of oral health adapted for dentistry by Locker (Fig. 1) from one proposed by the World Health Organisation for general health.[3] The model proposes that a hierarchy of impacts can arise

[1]*Senior Research Fellow,* [3]*Reader, Honorary Consultant,* [5]*Professor, Honorary Consultant; University of Dundee;* [2]*Senior Lecturer, University of Newcastle upon Tyne;* [4]*Lecturer, University of Birmingham*
Correspondence to: Dr Nigel Nuttall, DHSRU, Dundee Dental Hospital & School, Park Place, Dundee DD1 4HR
email: n.m.nuttall@dundee.ac.uk
REFEREED PAPER
Received 13.06.00; Accepted 31.07.00
© *British Dental Journal* 2001; **190:** 121–126

Table 1	Dimensions and the subjects of questions associated with them
Dimension	Subject of questions (two per dimension)
Functional limitation	Trouble pronouncing words, worsened taste
Physical pain	Aching in mouth, discomfort eating food
Psychological discomfort	Feeling self-concious or tense
Physical disability	Interrupted meals or poor diet
Psychological disability	Difficulty relaxing, embarrassment
Social disability	Irritability, difficulty in doing usual jobs
Handicap	Life less satisfying, inability to function

A guide to the UK adult dental health survey 1998

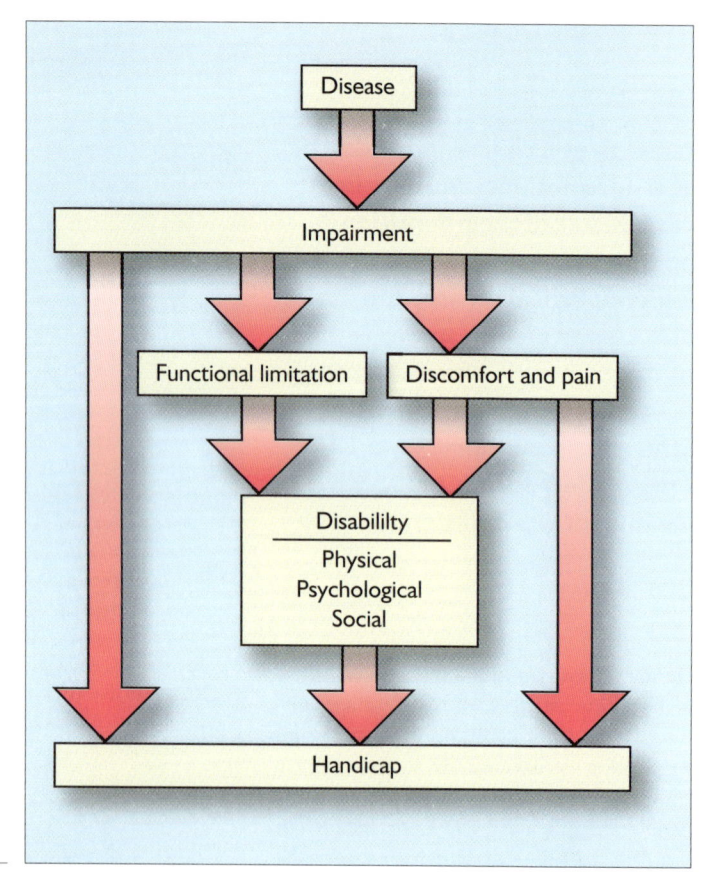

Fig. 1 Slade's formulation of Locker's conceptual model of oral health

important to people. Items were also added to cover what was expected to be the relatively rare occurrence of handicap which was not something that came out of the interviews but which were felt would be important to a few people according to Locker's model.

The original OHIP scale consisted of 49 questions organised into seven categories or dimensions. This long form of the OHIP scale would be suitable for use in clinical practice where a practitioner might want to establish an objective baseline against which to assess the impact of a course of dental care. A complex course of restorative treatment can be assessed on a variety of criteria from a technical point of view but it is less straightforward to assess the effect of it on a patient. One approach would be to ask the patient to complete the OHIP scale before and after treatment. This would get round the problems associated with direct questioning, where a patient may feel constrained about being objective with the dentist who has carried out the work, or where they may simply be unable to decide whether they feel any better than in the past.

A shorter version of the scale consisting of

from oral disease. For example, oral diseases can lead to the loss of teeth (impairment). At some stage this may lead to difficulties in chewing (functional limitation) or sometimes soreness brought on by dentures (discomfort). Eventually this may lead on to a restricted ability to eat or the need to avoid favourite foods (disability). In extreme cases this may even deter some people from eating anywhere outside the home or with their family members leading to a feeling of social isolation (handicap). In a sense the OHIP measure is a formalised and standardised equivalent to asking people from a dental point of view 'how have you been over the last year?'

The OHIP scale itself is a set of questions that were derived from in-depth interviews with people about how their oral condition affected their lives. Following this, the authors of the scale analysed the results to determine which factors were the most

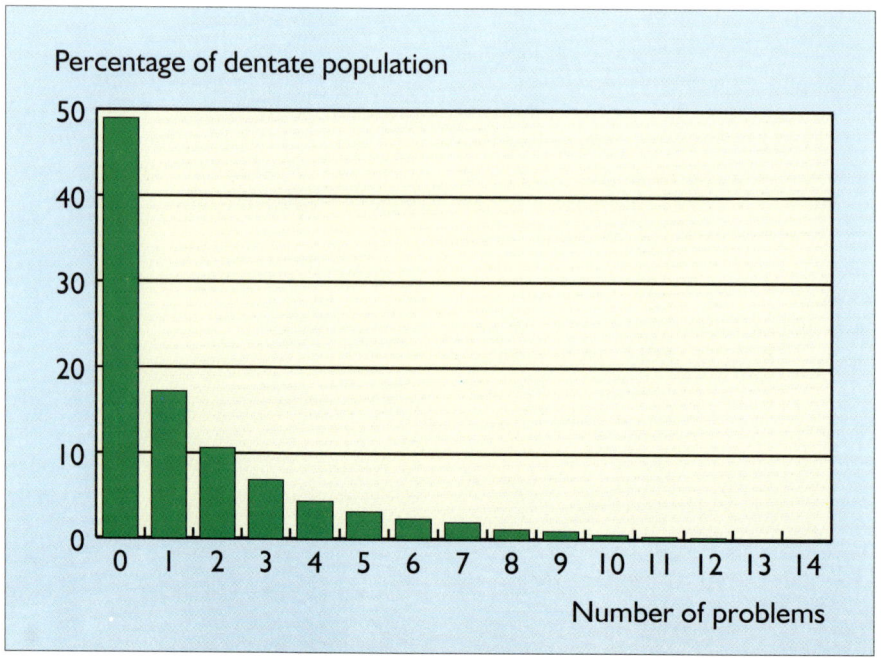

Fig. 2 Number of oral problems experienced by dentate adults in the UK in 1998

The impact of oral health

14 questions (2 for each dimension) was derived later on.[4] The dimensions and the subject of the questions associated with them are listed in Table 1.

Handicap for example was recorded in response to the questions such as *Have you found that life in general was less satisfying because of the condition of your teeth, mouth or gums?* and *Have you been totally unable to function because of the condition of your teeth mouth or gums?*

This shortened scale (OHIP-14) was the more practical to use in the context of the Adult Dental Health survey where many other questions needed to be asked. Shortening the scale does mean that some of the comprehensiveness of the original OHIP scale is lost, however, it still allows a basic overall measure of the impact of oral health on a national basis to be assessed.

How many people are affected by their oral condition?

The importance of the oral diseases as a factor that affects many people in their daily lives is shown by the finding that more than half of the population of the United Kingdom who had some natural teeth said their oral condition had affected them occasionally or more often over the preceding 12 months (Fig. 2). Most people said they only experienced one or two problems over the preceding year; nevertheless a sizable proportion (11.4%) experienced five or more forms of impact in the year preceding the survey.

What types of problem do people experience?

In Figure 3, the seven dimensions are ordered on the basis of how many dentate adults reported being affected by them. The questions underlying the dimensions are also summarised as short phrases. The most commonly experienced impact was pain (Fig. 3). Forty per cent of the dentate population reported being affected by oral pain occasionally or more often in the preceding 12 months. In the case of 3% of dentate adults, pain was experienced very often over the preceding year.

Many also felt that their oral state had a psychological effect on them in the sense that they felt self-conscious or felt tense (psychological discomfort) or that they found it difficult to relax or were embarrassed (psychological disability) about their oral condition. Over a quarter (27%) said they felt self-conscious or tense because of their oral condition and 18% said they felt embarrassed by their oral condition or that it made it difficult for them to relax.

Other impacts were experienced occasionally or more often during the preceding year by around 10% of adults; 10% said they had trouble pronouncing words or that their sense of taste had worsened (functional limitation); 9% said they had to interrupt meals or had an unsatisfactory diet (physical disability); 8% said they were irritable with others or had difficulty doing their usual jobs (social disability), and 8% said their life was less satisfying or that they were totally unable to function (handicap) because of their oral condition. The feeling of being totally unable to function as a result of their oral condition was a fairly rare experience and beyond the scope of the survey to

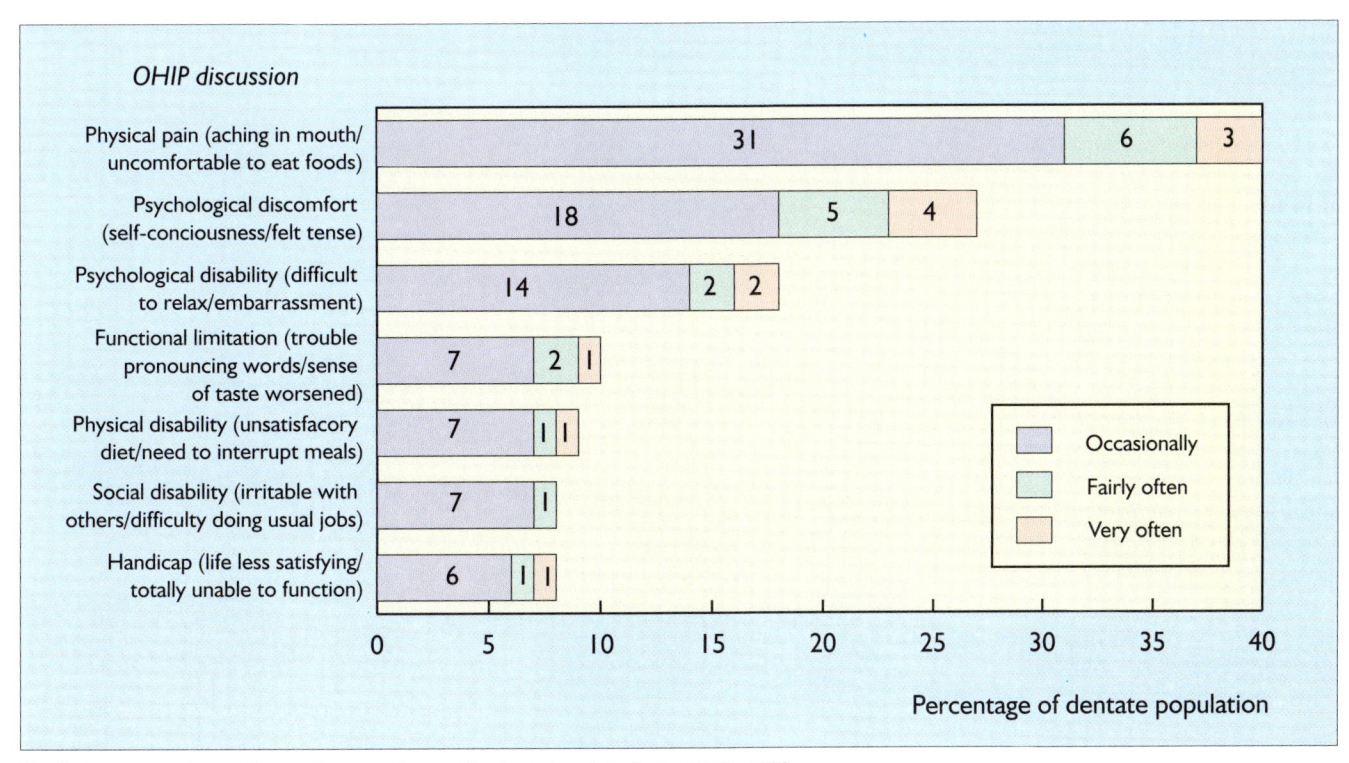

Fig. 3 Frequency of experience of types of impact by dentate adults in the UK in 1998

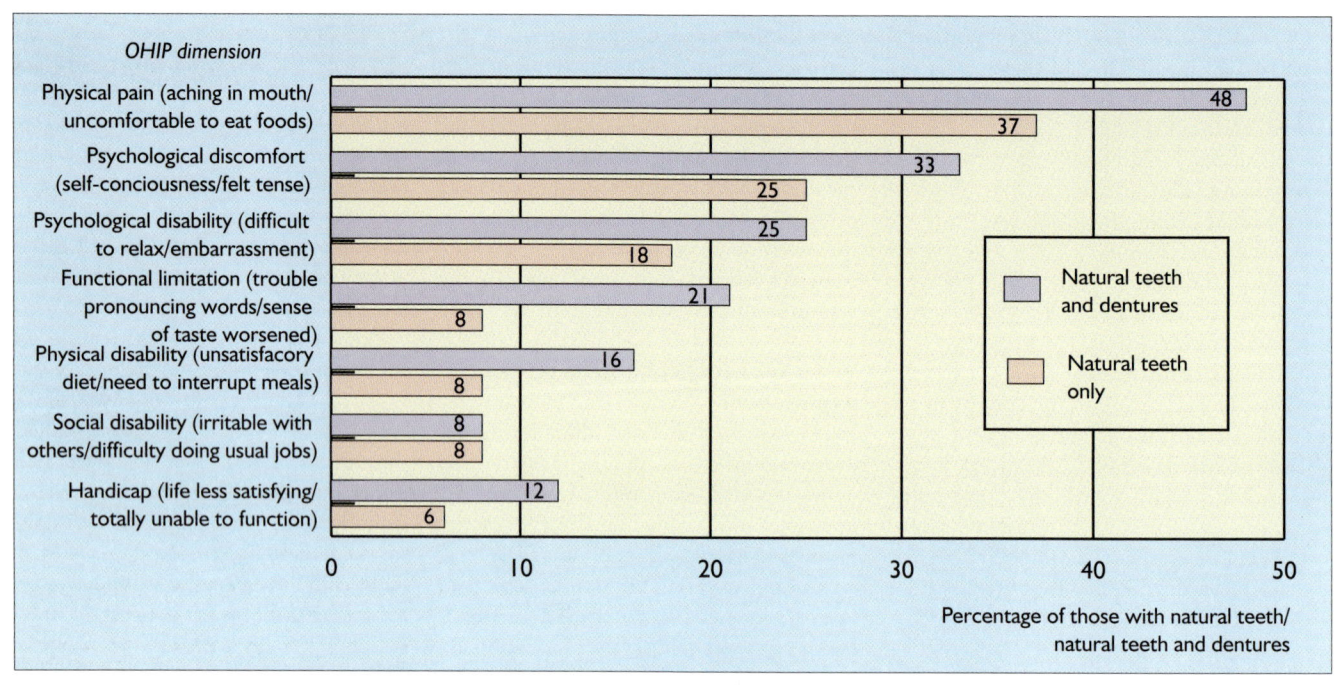

A guide to the UK adult dental health survey 1998

Fig. 4 The impact of oral health on people with natural teeth only or with natural teeth and some dentures

quantify reliably, nevertheless the finding that 76 people in the sample (1%) said this was an occasional experience over the preceding year suggests that oral condition can be a major determinant of reduced quality of life for a few people.

After pain the most frequently experienced problem were those categorised as psychological in nature. This is where people, for example, said they felt self-consciousness or found it difficult to relax as a result of their oral condition. Over a quarter of the dentate population said that they felt a form of psychological discomfort during the preceding year and 18% felt they had a problem that was in the category of a psychological disability. These results tend to suggest that issues concerned with aesthetics in dentistry affects quality of life more often (although not necessarily to the same degree) than issues of functionality in the dentate population as a whole.

Is a person's oral status associated with problems experienced?

The relationship between the perceived impact of oral condition and the clinical condition of the mouth is examined in Figures 4 and 5. People with dentures were

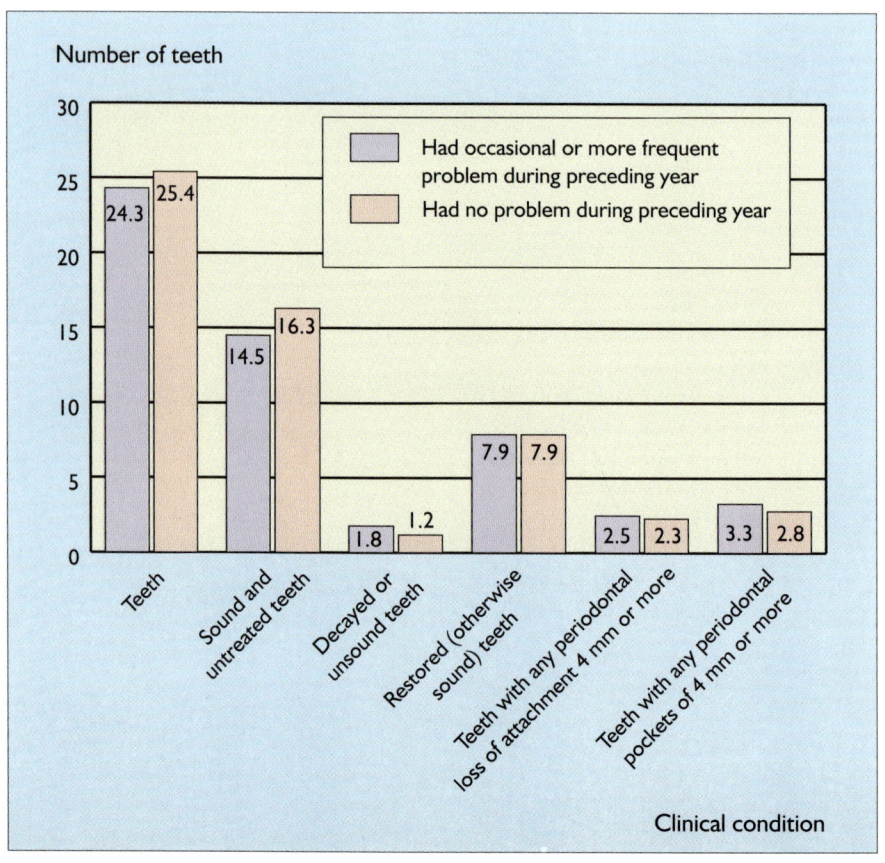

Fig. 5 The impact of oral health compared with aspects of the clinical condition of mouth

The impact of oral health

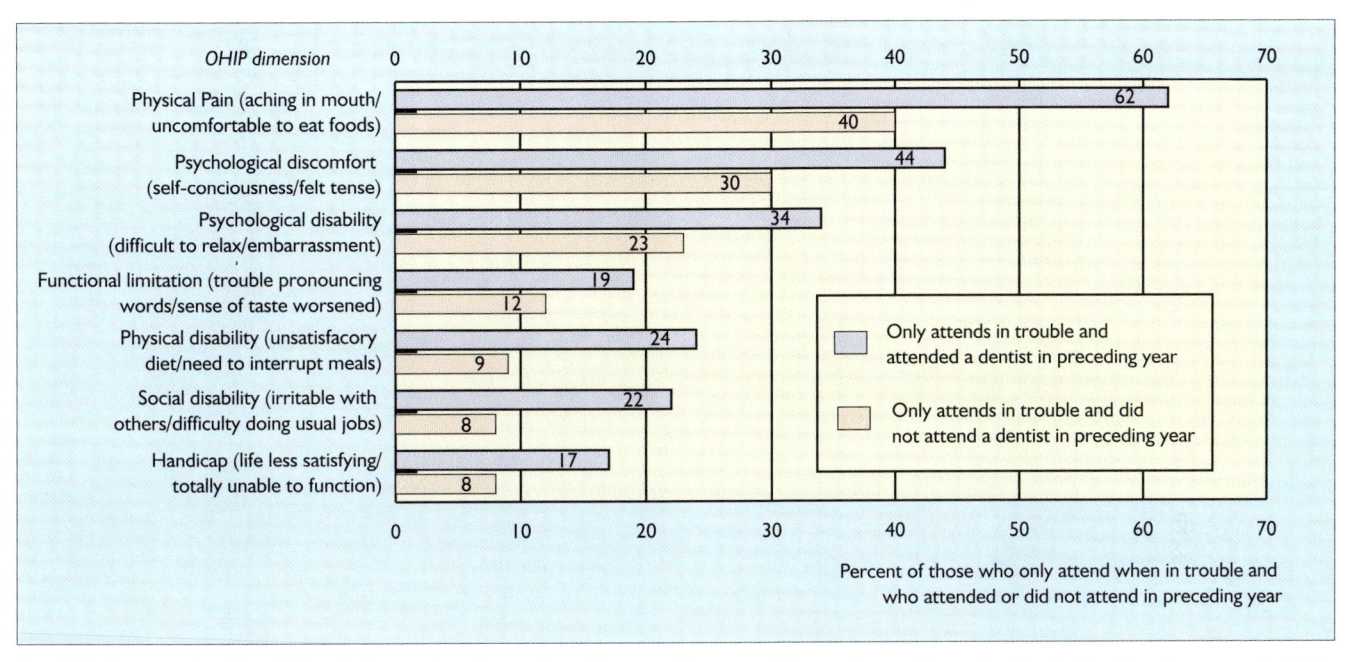

Fig. 6 The impact of oral health in relation to dental attendance in preceding year of those who say they only attend when they have some trouble with their teeth

more likely, than those with natural teeth only, to report having problems in six of the seven dimensions covered by the OHIP scale (Fig. 4). The main difference was in the experience of some form of functional limitation; 21% of those with dentures reported having this sort of problem compared with 8% of those who only had natural teeth. Denture wearers with some natural teeth were also twice as likely to say they had an unsatisfactory diet or trouble eating food (physical disability) than those with natural teeth only. They were also twice as likely as those with natural teeth only to say their oral condition made their life less satisfying or made them feel they were totally unable to function (handicap).

There was also a relationship between perceived impact and the clinical condition of a person's teeth but less so between impact and gum condition. Of the clinical indicators selected, those that were most markedly related to the experience of an OHIP-14 problem were the number of sound and the number of decayed teeth (Fig. 5). Those who reported an OHIP-14 problem had, on average, 1.8 decayed teeth and 14.5 sound teeth in comparison with an average of 1.2 decayed teeth and 16.3 sound teeth among those who did not report a problem.

Which OHIP-14 problems motivate people to go to the dentist?

Many people only attend a dentist when they have some trouble with their teeth. So what sort of problems covered by the OHIP-14 scale cause people who experience them to go to a dentist? The people who took part in this survey were asked if they usually went to a dentist for a regular check-up, an occasional check-up or only when they had some trouble with their teeth. They were also asked separately when they last visited a dentist. Figure 6 looks specifically at those who said they only go to see a dentist when they have some trouble with their teeth according to whether they visited in the preceding year or not and compares this with any OHIP problems they experienced over the preceding year.

People who say they usually put off attending for dental care until they have a problem and who attended in the year preceding the survey were more likely to have had experienced an OHIP-14 problem during that time. For example, 44% of those who only attend when having some dental trouble and who went to a dentist in the preceding year said they had felt self-conscious or tense as a result of their oral condition compared with 40% who did not go to a dentist. Nevertheless of those who only go to a dentist when they have a dental problem many did not go to a dentist despite having an OHIP-14 problem. Forty per cent of people who only attend when they have some tooth trouble did not attend despite having some dental pain in the preceding year and 8% said their oral condition made their life less satisfying or made them unable to function yet did not attend.

Is there any support for the model of oral health that OHIP-14 is based on?

A lot of the analysis of the OHIP-14 responses in the Adult Dental health survey has concerned itself with using the scale as a basic questionnaire to see what sort of problems people have with their teeth and gums. However, the scale is more than a standardised list of questions, it has an underlying model which sets out the way people's condition can affect them. It is beyond the scope of the Adult Dental Health survey to go in any depth into whether the results support the construction of the model underlying

A guide to the UK adult dental health survey 1998

the OHIP scale, however there is some support in the results for the scale conforming to the hierarchical nature of the model underlying it. The model views people as moving from one stage to another (Fig. 1); a person develops an impairment, which can sometimes become a functional limitation or discomfort. In some cases, although not all, this can then affect them in a psychological or social way and may eventually, if severe enough, become a handicap. It would thus be expected that more people would be affected by functional limitation, discomfort or pain than by physical, psychological or social disability and fewer still would be affected by handicap. The results bear out this prediction by and large, with pain and psychological discomfort being the most frequently reported problems; social physical and psychological disability being in the middle of the order; and handicap being the least frequently experienced problem.

How many people are handicapped by oral disease?

In the most severe cases the model of oral health on which OHIP-14 is based (Fig. 1) suggests that some people can become handicapped by their oral condition. In addition to revealing just how often people can be affected by the types of problem considered by the OHIP scale some consideration should also be given to the more rare occurrences that were revealed. There is a limit to the accuracy of these surveys for predicting the prevalence of rare conditions in the population. Use of the findings concerning how many people occasionally felt totally unable to cope as a result of their oral condition would be an example of this. Nevertheless, the finding that 76 out of over 6,000 people felt sufficiently bad about their oral condition that it occasionally made them feel totally unable to cope indicates the level of severity of impact that oral conditions can have on some people. This will reflect the sum of a variety of specific clinical conditions, nevertheless, it suggests that somewhere around 1% of the population may consider themselves severely affected by their oral condition. The knock-on effects of this finding need to be considered further. Potentially there are far reaching considerations such the extent to which these conditions affect activities such as work and even the extent that they might put pressure on mental health services.

What has the OHIP-14 measure revealed about the impact of oral health on adults?

The findings show that people can be affected in different ways by their oral condition and that for some the impact can be sufficiently serious that their lives are affected. Physical pain and the psychological impact of oral conditions were the most frequently reported problems that affected people. However, sight must not be lost of the very severe impact that oral condition can have on some people to the extent that they feel totally unable to cope. This cannot readily be appreciated simply from knowledge of the clinical conditions that exist in a population. There is a need for dentists and dental epidemiologists to consider how people live with their oral health state through the use of measures such as OHIP in order to appreciate where a person is so adversely affected by their dental condition that they are handicapped by it.

This article has been refereed under the British Dental Journal reviewing process. Full details of sample numbers and the criteria for the clinical examinations can be found in the survey report. We would like to acknowledge the work of Alison Walker, Maureen Kelly and other staff of the Office for National Statistics. This work was undertaken by a consortium comprising the Office for National Statistics and the Dental Schools of the Universities of Birmingham, Dundee, Newcastle and Wales who received funding from the United Kingdom Health Departments; the views expressed in this publication are those of the authors and not necessarily those of the Health Departments nor of the other members of the consortium. Nigel Nuttall acknowledges support from the Chief Scientist Office of the Scottish Executive who do not necessarily share the views expressed.

1. Kelly M, Steele J, Nuttall N, Bradnock G, Morris J, Nunn J, Pine C, Pitts N, Treasure E, White D. *Adult Dental Health Survey - Oral Health in the United Kingdom 1998.* London: The Stationery Office 2000.
2. Slade G (ed). *Measuring oral health and quality of life.* Chapel Hill: University of North Carolina, Dental Ecology 1997.
3. Locker D. Measuring oral health a conceptual framework. *Community Dent Health* 1988; 5: 5-13.
4. Slade G D. Derivation and validation of a short form oral health impact profile. *Community Dentistry Oral Epidemiol* 1997; 25: 284-290.

Dental attendance in 1998 and implications for the future

N. M. Nuttall,[1] G. Bradnock,[2] D. White,[3] J. Morris,[4] and J. Nunn,[5]

The 1998 survey of Adult Dental Health in the UK was carried out under the auspices of the Office of National Statistics together with the Universities of Birmingham, Dundee, Newcastle-upon-Tyne and Wales. A key behavioural indicator in these decennial surveys is whether people say they go to a dentist for a regular dental check-up, an occasional dental check-up or only when they have trouble with their teeth. The proportion of dentate adults in the UK who report attending for regular dental check-ups has risen from 43% in 1978 to 59% in 1998. Older adults (over 55 years old) in 1998 were the most likely to say they attend for regular dental check-ups. Many younger adults (16–24) in 1998 said they went to a dentist less often than 5 years previously, they were also the least likely to say they attend for regular dental check-ups. Dental anxiety remains a problem for many dental patients but another factor of importance to many is their want to be involved in the treatment process and especially to be given an estimate of treatment costs.

In brief
- The proportion of dentate adults in the UK who report attending for regular dental check-ups has risen from 43% in 1978 to 59% in 1998.
- Dentate adults over 55 in 1998 were the most likely to say they attend for regular check-ups, the proportion of them reporting this has more than doubled over the last 20 years.
- Almost a half (48%) of 16–24 years old in 1998 said they went to a dentist less frequently than they used to, they were also the least likely to say they attend for regular dental check-ups.
- A half of dentate adults said they would like to be given an estimate of treatment costs without commitment.
- The most frequent reason given for not attending for check-ups among those who only go when they have trouble with their teeth is that they do not see the point in visiting unless they have to.

[1]Senior Research Fellow, University of Dundee
[2]Senior Lecturer [3]Lecturer [4]Lecturer, University of Birmingham [5]Senior Lecturer, University of Newcastle upon Tyne
Correspondence to: Dr Nigel Nuttall, DHSRU, Dundee Dental Hospital & School, Park Place, Dundee DD1 4HR
email: n.m.nuttall@dundee.ac.uk
REFEREED PAPER
Received 13.06.00; Accepted 31.07.00
© British Dental Journal 2001; 190: 177–182

The national surveys of Adult Dental Health have given a 10-yearly summary of the clinical condition of adults in the United Kingdom on three previous occasions. The fourth report in the series was published in March of 2000. For the 1998 survey 4,984 addresses were identified at which all adults over 16 in residence were asked to take part in the survey; 21% of households refused and no contact was made at 5% of them. In total, 6,204 adults were interviewed following which those with some teeth were asked to undergo a dental examination; 3,817 (72%) of those eligible agreed. A weighting system based on some of the interview responses of those who consented to be dentally examined and those who were interviewed but not dentally examined was used to reduce bias from non-response.[1] The survey was carried out under the auspices of the Office of National Statistics together with the Universities of

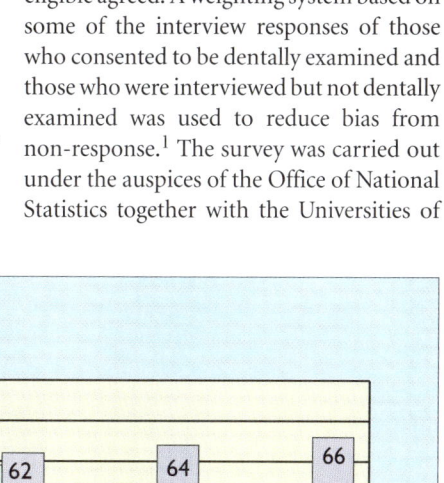

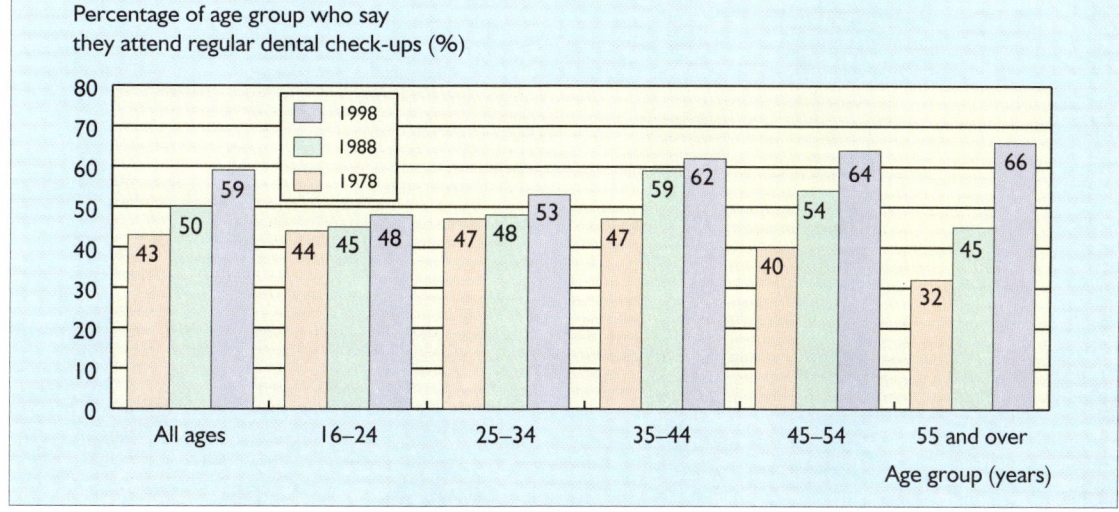

Fig. 1 Dentate adults who say their usual reason for attending a dentist is for regular dental check-ups in the UK and by age group 1978–1998

Age group	1978	1988	1998
All ages	43	50	59
16–24	44	45	48
25–34	47	48	53
35–44	47	59	62
45–54	40	54	64
55 and over	32	45	66

A guide to the UK adult dental health survey 1998

Birmingham, Dundee, Newcastle-upon-Tyne and Wales.

A key behavioural indicator that has been used since the first survey of adult dental health of England and Wales in 1968 is whether people say they go to a dentist for a regular dental check-up, an occasional dental check-up or only when they have trouble with their teeth. Self-assessed dental attendance has been shown to have clear associations with dental health. The 1998 survey shows that those who say they attend only when they have some trouble with their teeth had one less tooth on average than those who attend for regular check-ups.[1] In addition the condition of these teeth was less satisfactory on the whole; those who only attend when they have some trouble with their teeth were, in 1998, twice as likely to have some active decay and six times more likely to have some unrestorable caries than those who say they go for regular dental check-ups.[1]

This article looks at the reported dental attendance behaviour of the dentate United Kingdom population and what the 1998 Adult Dental Health survey reveals about the reasons why people who have some natural teeth visit a dentist, what they mean when they say they for regular dental check-ups and what puts people off going to a dentist.

Did more dentate adults in the UK in 1998 say they go for regular dental check-ups than in the past?
The proportion of the UK population who say they usually attend for regular dental check-ups has risen from 43% in 1978 to 59% in 1998 (Fig. 1). This growth in attending for regular dental check-ups has been largely among people aged 35 and over. Among those aged 16–24 there has only been a 4% growth in the uptake of regular dental check-ups, with a similar level (6%) among 25–34 year olds over 20 years. Furthermore 15% more of those aged between 35–44 and 24% more of those aged over 45–54 in 1998 said they usually went for regular check-ups in comparison with 1978. The most marked change in seeking dental check-ups was among dentate adults aged 55 and over which has more than doubled over

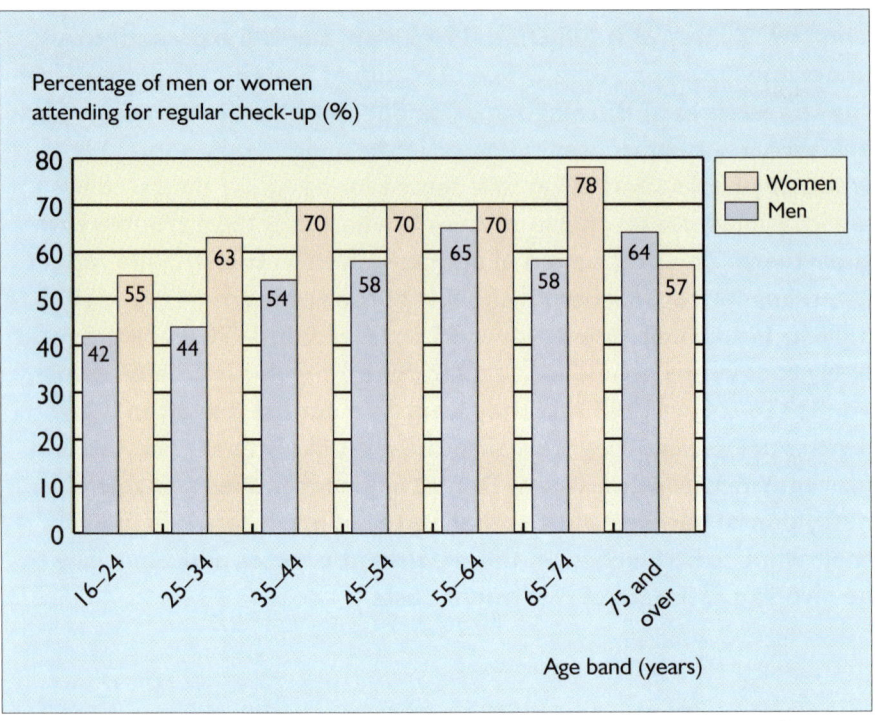

Fig. 2 The percentage of men or women who say they usually attend for regular dental check-ups by age group

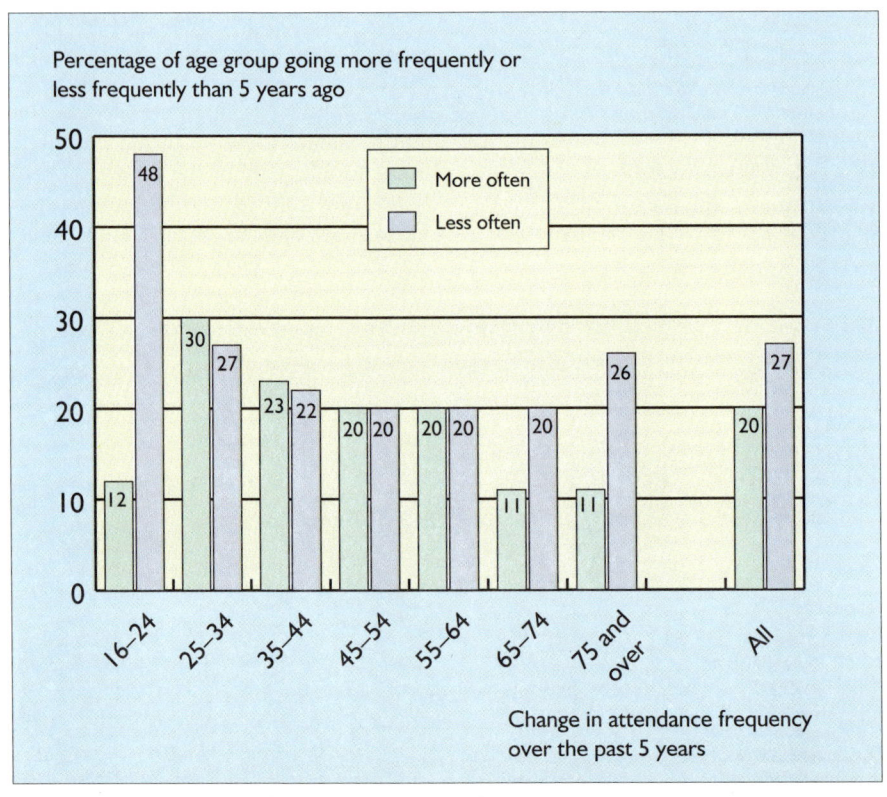

Fig. 3 Change in attendance frequency over 5 years by age group

Dental attendance

the past 20 years, and who in 1998 were the age-group who were the most likely to say they sought regular dental check-ups

What are the characteristics of dentate adults who say they go for regular check-ups?

Dental attendance behaviour is markedly related to age and gender. Men of all ages were less likely to go for dental check-ups than women, except among those aged over 75 (Fig. 2). Those least likely to go for regular dental check-ups were young men; fewer than a half of men aged below 34 said they went for regular dental check-ups. So why should older people be more likely to seek regular dental check-ups than the young? One factor may be that older people change their behaviour, perhaps in response to greater perceived need or through having more disposable income in general than the young. However a competing explanation is not that people change their behaviour as they get older but that the least dentally healthy progressively drop out of the dentate population by losing all their teeth leaving mainly those with 'good' dental habits in older age groups. This latter possibility may be a partial explanation but the rate of loss of people through edentulousness[2] is lower than the rate of increase in uptake of regular check-ups, which suggests that some of the improvement is also occurring because of people changing their attendance behaviour, as they get older.

Do people say they go to a dentist more or less often than they used to?

Although more people now say they go for regular check-ups than in the past, more people also reported that they went less often to a dentist than they did 5 years previously (Fig. 3). Only in one age group (25–34 year olds) did more people say they went more often than less often in comparison with 5 years before. The most marked drop-off was among the young; almost a half (48%) of 16–24 year olds said they attended a dentist less often by 1998 than they did 5 years previously. Overall, 7% of the population said they went to a dentist less often in 1998 in comparison with 5 years previously.

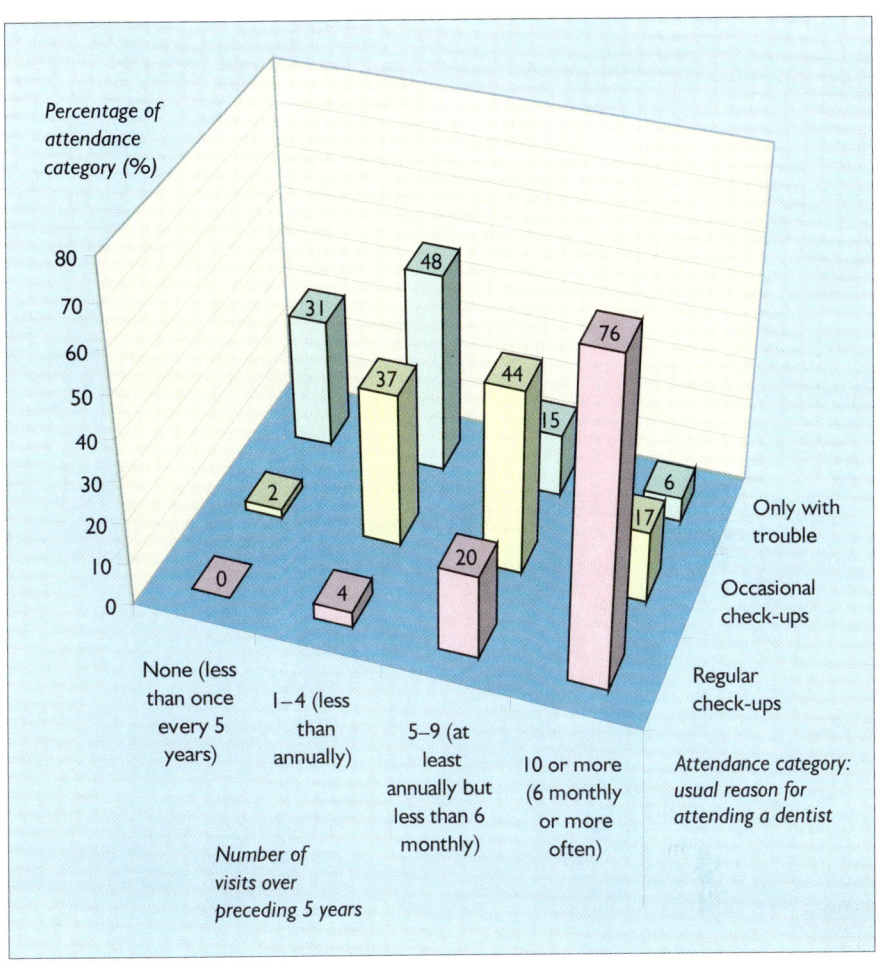

Fig. 4 Self-reported frequency of dental attendance compared with usual reason for attending

These results seem to be giving conflicting indications about what is happening to dental attendance. More dentate adults say they are going for regular dental check-ups yet more also say they now visit a dentist less often than they did 5 years ago. A large part of the apparent contradiction stems from the amount of change occurring among those aged 16 to 24. Many of these adults will be comparing their current attendance with that when they were under 18 and reflect the change that occurs as people enter adulthood. Potential reasons may include the cost of dental treatment but the 1998 survey has shown that people in the 16 to 24-year-old age group were actually the age-group who were least likely to say they find NHS dental treatment expensive[1] (although this may reflect the lack of experience of NHS dental costs as a result of having last attended when they were aged 18 or under and therefore exempt from contributing to costs). A revealing finding from the survey was that 53% of those who in the past used to go for regular check-ups, but no longer do so, said that they had no choice about going for regular check-ups in the past, which suggests that coercion is not a particularly effective way of building a habit of regular attendance.[1]

What is a regular dental attender?

The term regular attender has slipped from the Adult Dental Health surveys into the dental lexicon without much challenge despite its meaning being far from clear in terms of whether it refers to regularity or frequency of attendance (eg 6 monthly) or the underlying motivation for attendance

A guide to the UK adult dental health survey 1998

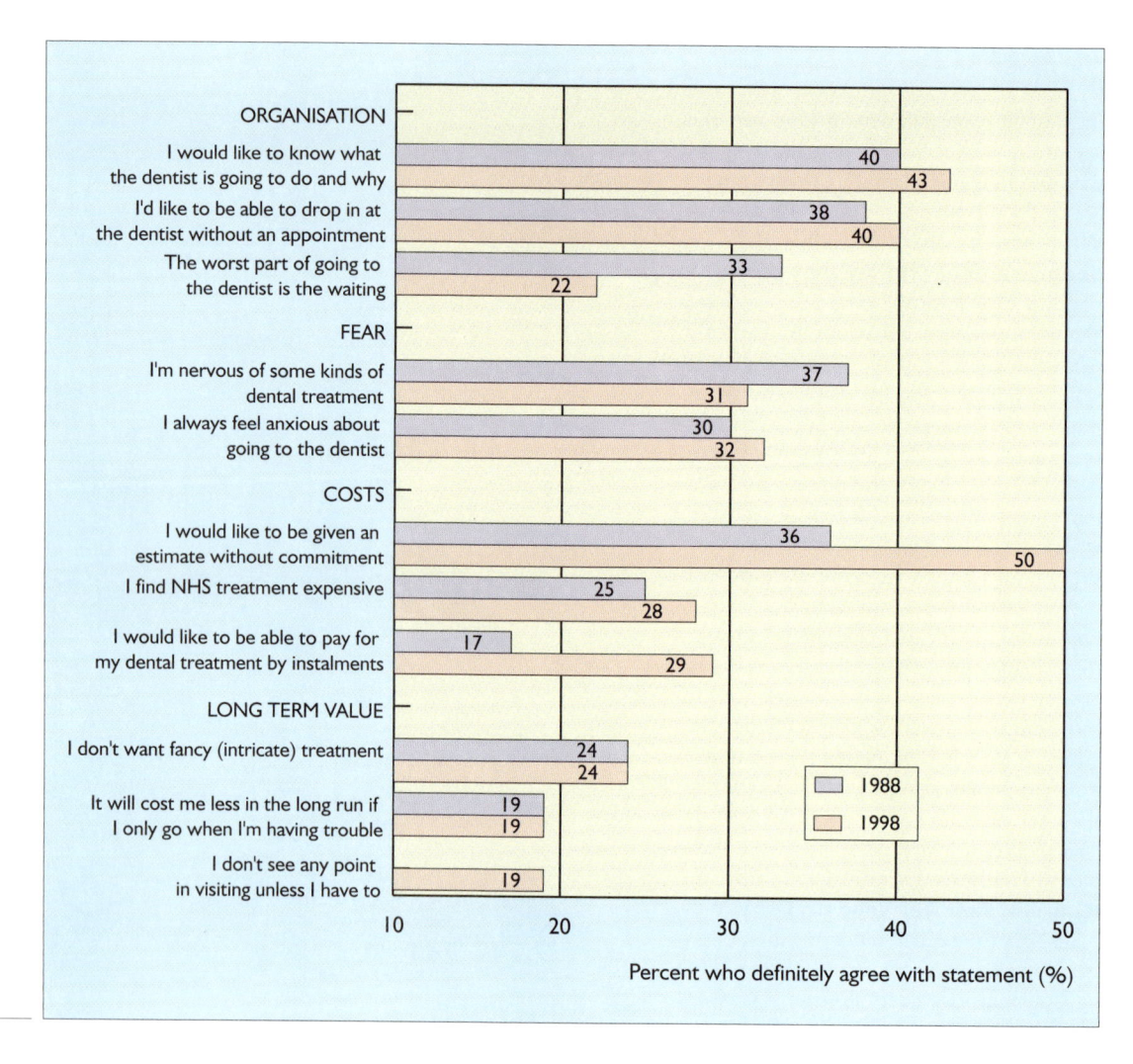

Fig. 5 Feelings about going to the dentist, 1988–1998

Statement	1988	1998
ORGANISATION		
I would like to know what the dentist is going to do and why	40	43
I'd like to be able to drop in at the dentist without an appointment	38	40
The worst part of going to the dentist is the waiting	33	22
FEAR		
I'm nervous of some kinds of dental treatment	37	31
I always feel anxious about going to the dentist	30	32
COSTS		
I would like to be given an estimate without commitment	36	50
I find NHS treatment expensive	25	28
I would like to be able to pay for my dental treatment by instalments	17	29
LONG TERM VALUE		
I don't want fancy (intricate) treatment	24	24
It will cost me less in the long run if I only go when I'm having trouble	19	19
I don't see any point in visiting unless I have to		19

Percent who definitely agree with statement (%)

(usually visiting without symptoms to check everything is alright).

For the 1998 Adult Dental Health survey we felt that some attempt should be made to determine what people actually meant when they replied to the question which asked 'In general do you attend for a regular check-up, an occasional check-up or only when you have some trouble with your teeth'. So the people who took part were asked how often they had attended over the past 5 years in order to get an indication of how often they went to a dentist. This was particularly revealing; three-quarters of those who said they went for regular dental check-ups said they had gone to a dentist 10 or more times over the preceding 5 years (usually the exact figure of 10 times in 5 years was mentioned), which is equivalent to a 6-monthly interval (Fig. 4).

The '6-monthly dental visit' is a popular concept of what constitutes the most appropriate interval to leave between dental visits and still seems to hold sway among patients, at least as that which constitutes the frequency that is appropriate for 'regular dental check-ups'. Yet the evidence base for the recommendation has been called into doubt. A committee of dentists looked into the scientific basis of dental health education[3] and concluded that: 'there is little evidence to support a specific interval or to quantify its benefit' despite going on to suggest the maximum period between oral examinations for everyone, irrespective of age or dental condition, should be 1 year. The experience in Scotland of a longitudinally monitored sample of dentate adults suggests that going to a dentist every 6 months, without lapse or delay over a 5-year period is actually extremely rare even if a 3-month leeway is allowed for difficulties in scheduling.[4] Even consistent annual dental visits are less than usual.[5] If anything dental attendance often seems more likely to go in 'bursts' of visits over a period followed by a longer than usual lapse.[5] It may be that people say they attend every 6 months because this is congruent with their description of themselves as 'regular dental attenders' and some may even be unaware that their actual behaviour is often less consistent or less frequent.

The data in Figure 4 show there is a clear difference in reported attendance frequency between those who say they attend for regular check-ups and those who wait until they have some trouble with their teeth. Three-quarters of 'regular attenders' (76%) said they visited a dentist once every 6 months over the preceding 5 years and about the same proportion (79%) of those who only went when they had some trouble with their teeth said they went less

Dental attendance

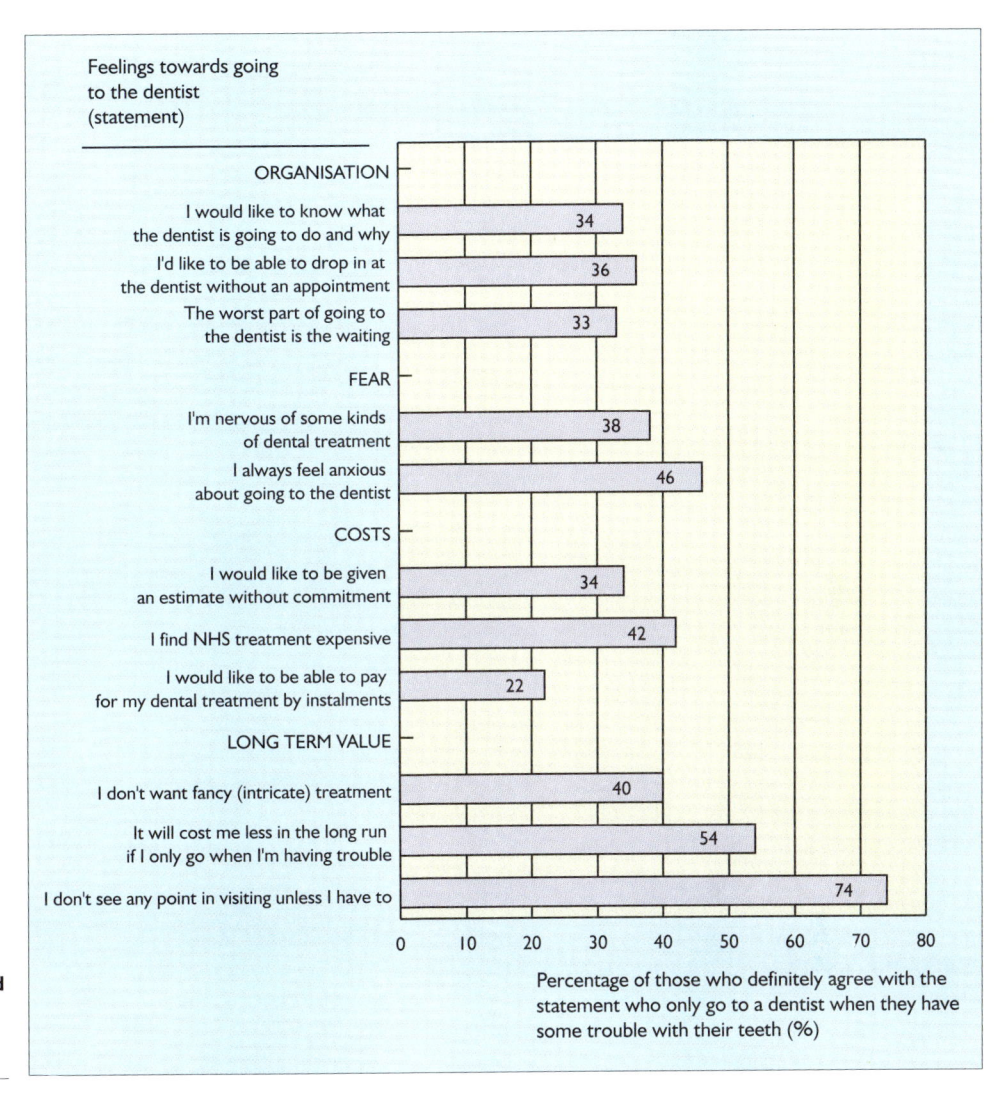

Fig. 6 Those who say they only attend when they have some trouble with their teeth against feelings towards going to the dentist

[Chart: Feelings towards going to the dentist (statement) — Percentage of those who definitely agree with the statement who only go to a dentist when they have some trouble with their teeth (%)]

ORGANISATION
- I would like to know what the dentist is going to do and why: 34
- I'd like to be able to drop in at the dentist without an appointment: 36
- The worst part of going to the dentist is the waiting: 33

FEAR
- I'm nervous of some kinds of dental treatment: 38
- I always feel anxious about going to the dentist: 46

COSTS
- I would like to be given an estimate without commitment: 34
- I find NHS treatment expensive: 42
- I would like to be able to pay for my dental treatment by instalments: 22

LONG TERM VALUE
- I don't want fancy (intricate) treatment: 40
- It will cost me less in the long run if I only go when I'm having trouble: 54
- I don't see any point in visiting unless I have to: 74

than once a year. However, what people mean when they use the terms is still not entirely clear as 30% of those who said they only go when they have some trouble with their teeth said their previous visit was for a dental check-up.[1]

What puts off those who avoid going to the dentist?

Fear and anxiety is the most usual reaction that is popularly referred to when the topic of dentists or dental visits are brought up. The reasons why people avoid going to a dentist was the subject of research in the 1980s in which people were interviewed to find out what put them off going to a dentist.[6] The issues people mentioned led to the development of a set of questions that were included in the 1988 and 1998 surveys. Principal components factor analysis was used to examine the relationships between the responses to each statement.[1] This confirmed that the statements related to different aspects of going to the dentist and identified four factors which could be used to group the statements: fear; cost; the value of dental treatment and going to the dentist; and the organisational aspects of going to the dentist.

What people seemed most concerned about were issues to do with the cost of dental treatment (Fig. 5); 50% said they would like to be given an estimate of the cost of dental treatment without commitment. In many cases this seems to be a different concern from the expensiveness of treatment as such, because many fewer dentate adults (28%) said they found NHS dental treatment expensive or would like to pay for their care by instalments (29%). This may suggest that many people feel they would like to be more involved in the planning of their treatment. This might also be implicit in the next most frequent response where 43% said they definitely felt they would like 'to know what the dentist is doing and why'. Furthermore when people were asked to rank the statements they had identified as agreeing with most strongly 'knowing what the dentist is doing' came top of the list.[1] The statement probably applies more to operative procedures rather than treatment planning, nevertheless taken together the responses suggest that many people feel uninvolved in the process of their dental treatment. People want to know 'how much?' and 'what's going on'.

A guide to the UK adult dental health survey 1998

When the new General Dental Services contract was introduced in 1990 there was a requirement that patients should be provided with estimates for dental treatment planned. The regulations were relaxed after a couple of years but are still largely in place for certain circumstances and still require that a patient who asks for an estimate be given one.[7] It seems very likely that many patients do not know about this entitlement at present and yet would clearly welcome the opportunity if they knew it existed. Furthermore, we must also not lose sight that 'without commitment' ought to mean allowing a person to go away and consider a treatment proposal. Both of these findings give an unsettling indication that many patients currently feel they are not in control of what happens to them in dental surgeries.

The issue of access to healthcare is high on the political agenda at the moment with Government statements about the provision of walk-in dental clinics and the intention to encourage late opening medical and dental surgeries. It is certainly an aspect that the people who took part in the survey were interested in; 40% said they would like to be able to drop in at the dentist without an appointment.

Significantly fewer people in 1998 felt that the worst part of going to the dentist was the waiting in comparison with 1988. This is intriguing as it might mean waiting for dental care is less common now than in 1988 or that other aspects of dental visits have taken over as being the 'worst' thing about going to the dentist.

Fear and anxiety is clearly a problem for many but was mentioned by fewer people than information issues. About a third of dentate adults definitely agreed that they always feel anxious about going to the dentist. However, we must be clear that this does not tell us anything about the relative impact of fear and anxiety that probably has more intensity and more impact as a feeling than has wanting information.

The factors which were mentioned least often as affecting people in general were those classified as concerning the long-term value of attending for dental care; 24% definitely agreed that 'I don't want fancy (intricate) treatment', 19% agreed that 'it will cost me more in the long run if I only go when I'm having some trouble with my teeth' in both the 1988 and the 1998 surveys. A similar proportion (19%) agreed with a new statement introduced into the 1998 survey that "I don't see the point in visiting unless I have to'.

However, although fewest people overall agreed with these statements about long-term value they were nevertheless the statements that most strongly differentiated between regular and in trouble attenders (Fig. 6). People who agreed they could not see the point in visiting a dentist unless they had to were far more likely only to attend when they had some trouble with their teeth (74%) than seek regular dental check-ups (20%). Furthermore many are fearful about going to a dentist and find dental treatment expensive but this does not necessarily put them off attending for check-ups; people who said they were anxious were equally as likely to say they went for regular check-ups (43%) as to say they only attend when having some trouble with their teeth (46%).

What has the 1998 Adult Dental Health survey told us about dental patients views about visiting the dentist?

The overall picture that the 1998 survey has given us about adult dental attendance behaviour is that many people abandon regular check-ups in early adulthood, often because there seems to be no clear value to them in seeking regular dental check-ups, but many then appear to begin to see some benefit to check-ups, as they get older.

Most people who describe themselves as going for regular dental check-ups also said they attended on a 6-monthly basis over the past 5 years despite recommendations that an annual visit is sufficient for most healthy adults.[3]

Recent pronouncements suggest that Governmental policy on the NHS is being directed at providing a modern health service that meets the expressed needs of patients. The 1998 survey tends to suggest that patients would indeed welcome some of these plans, such as the provision of drop-in clinics. Another concern among dental patients is that they want to have more information about their dental care; such as wanting to know, without obligation, what their treatment is going to cost them and what their dentist is doing during treatment. This suggests many people feel they are not in full control of what happens to them in dental surgeries. The dental profession should give urgent consideration about how to address this, as knowing what something is going to cost and what is going to be done to them seem perfectly reasonable things for patients to be informed about.

1. Kelly M, Steele J, Nuttall N, Bradnock G, Morris J, Nunn J, Pine C, Pitts N, Treasure E, White D. *Adult Dental Health Survey – Oral Health in the United Kingdom 1998.* London: The Stationery Office 2000. (Table 2.2.9, Table 3.1.23, Table 6.1.9, Table 6.1.10, Table 6.2.3 & Table 6.1.8).
2. Steele J, Treasure E, Pitts N B, Morris J, Bradnock G. Tooth loss in the United Kingdom in 1998 and implications for the future. *Br Dent J* 2000; **189**; 598-603.
3. *Health Education Authority, The Scientific Basis of Dental Health Education (Fourth Edition).* London; HEA, 1996.
4. Eddie S. Frequency of dental attendance in the General Dental Service in Scotland; a comparison with claimed attendance. *Br Dent J* 1984; **157**: 267-270.
5. Nuttall N M, Davies J A. The frequency of dental attendance of Scottish dentate adults between 1978 and 1988. *Br Dent J* 1991; **171**: 161-165.
6. Finch H, Keegan J, Ward K, Senyal Sen B S. *Barriers to the receipt of dental care.* London: Social & Community Planning Research, 1988.
7. Management Executive Letter. General Dental Services. Relaxation of the requirement to issue treatment plans. *NHS Management Executive,* January 1992.

This article has been refereed under the British Dental Journal reviewing process. Full details of sample numbers and the criteria for the clinical examinations can be found in the survey report. We would like to acknowledge the work of Alison Walker, Maureen Kelly and other staff of the Office for National Statistics. This work was undertaken by a consortium comprising the Office for National Statistics and the Dental Schools of the Universities of Birmingham, Dundee, Newcastle and Wales who received funding from the United Kingdom Health Departments; the views expressed in this publication are those of the authors and not necessarily those of the Health Departments nor of the other members of the consortium. Nigel Nuttall acknowledges support from the Chief Scientist Office of the Scottish Executive who do not necessarily share the views expressed.

Dental attitudes and behaviours in 1998 and implications for the future

G. Bradnock,[1] D. A. White,[2] N. M. Nuttall,[3] A. J. Morris,[4] E. T. Treasure,[5] and C. M. Pine,[6]

The 1998 Adult Dental Health Survey included face to face interviews with participants to determine their dental attitudes and behaviours. This article considers reported oral hygiene practices, treatment choices, satisfaction with appearance of teeth, attitudes towards wearing dentures and how these have changed since previous surveys. Although overall there has been a steady improvement in dental health attitudes, adults from disadvantaged households are still lagging behind. This has implications for social equity.

A face-to-face interview, conducted in the home by ONS interviewers, has always formed the backbone of the decennial studies into adult dental health. Over the years questions have been asked concerning what choices people would make about their oral health should they be faced with making a decision. Some questions relate to choices around visiting the dentist and others are about the choices of treatment available to them. Attitudes related to reported dental attendance are examined in a companion paper in this series.[1] This paper looks at the reported oral hygiene practices of respondents, what choices they said that they would make in certain circumstances, their satisfaction with the appearance of their teeth, their attitudes towards the possibility of wearing dentures in the future and individual concerns expressed.

When the first adult dental health study of England and Wales was undertaken in 1968, 37% of adults were reported as edentate. In 1998 that appalling statistic has reduced to 12% in England and Wales and 13% in the UK. A further analysis of tooth loss can be found in a companion paper in this series.[2] The dramatic changes in oral health over the last 40 years are partly the result of changes in attitude towards self-care and dental treatment. However, these same changes are also a factor in changing expectations and attitudes.

A series of questions were asked in the 1998 interview to investigate oral health behaviour and attitudes (Fig. 1). The 1998 responses to these questions are related to previous decades to establish whether attitudes have changed, with a view to determining the implications for the future of dental care. The basic oral health messages are now well embedded, in some form or

---

[1]*Senior Lecturer in Dental Public Health,* [2]*Lecturer in Oral Health,* [4]*Lecturer in Dental Public Health, School of Dentistry, The University of Birmingham;* [3]*Senior Research Fellow,* [6]*Reader in Dental Public Health, Head of Section of Dental Public Health & Health Psychology, Dundee Dental School;* [5]*Professor of Dental Public Health, University of Wales College of Medicine*
e-mail: g.marchment@bham.ac.uk
REFEREED PAPER
Received 13.06.00; Accepted 31.07.00
© British Dental Journal 2001; 190: 228–232

Fig. 1   Questions from the interview relating to oral hygiene, treatment preferences, appearance of teeth and attitudes towards dentures

Oral hygiene

Do you usually keep your top/bottom plate in at night?
How often do you clean your teeth nowadays?
Do you use anything other than an ordinary toothbrush and toothpaste for dental hygiene purposes? If yes, what do you use?
Has a dentist or any of the dental staff demonstrated to you how to clean your teeth?

Treatment preferences

If you went to the dentist with an aching back tooth, would you prefer the dentist to take it out or fill it, supposing it could be filled?
If the dentist said a front/back tooth would have to be extracted (taken out) or crowned, what would you prefer?

Appearance

In general, how do you feel about the appearance of your teeth (and/or dentures), are you satisfied or not satisfied with the way they look?
If not, what is it about the way your teeth or dentures look that makes you not satisfied?

Dentures

Do you find the thought of losing all your own teeth and having full dentures very upsetting, a little upsetting or not at all upsetting?
Do you find the thought of having a partial denture to replace some of your teeth very upsetting, a little upsetting or not at all upsetting?

NB This is a digest of questions asked in the survey.
For full details see reference 3.

A guide to the UK adult dental health survey 1998

another, in the folklore of the UK community. Phrases such as 'if you don't look after your teeth, you will lose them' are well known. Thus if people have some concerns about their future dental progress this may be reflected in the oral hygiene practices they claim to adopt.

What oral hygiene behaviour do people report?

A growing emphasis toward aesthetic considerations both in the media and dental practice is being demonstrated, therefore questions related to satisfaction with appearance can be considered as one barometer of oral health. Reported oral hygiene practices also reflect the level to which the UK population is receiving oral hygiene advice. Of those dentate adults questioned, 74% reported cleaning their teeth at least once a day. This comprised 83% of women and 64% of men. Figure 2 shows how this reported behaviour has changed since 1978. Amongst adults who claim to only attend the dentist when they have trouble, the proportion indicating that they brush at least twice a day has increased from 49% in 1978 to 61% in 1998. This is a rise of 12% compared with only a 2% rise amongst reported regular attenders.

Amongst those who wore dentures, over half reported wearing their denture at night, in conflict with current dental advice.

Figure 3 shows changes in the reported use of oral hygiene products since 1978. Whereas in 1978 almost 80% claimed to only use a toothbrush and toothpaste, 20 years later we can demonstrate that over 20% now indicate use of floss and/or a mouthwash in addition to toothbrushing. There was a clear indication that those from non-manual backgrounds were more likely than those from manual backgrounds to report using such additional methods. As these data are essentially interview responses, actual usage can only be estimated. It is possible that those from the non-manual backgrounds are more aware of alternative forms of oral hygiene and are probably more able to purchase floss and mouthrinses than those in lower income brackets. However the increased attention given to extra oral hygiene aids such as floss and mouthrinses in both professional and commercial campaigns at least makes people aware of what they should be using. It is interesting to note however that 38% of respondents cannot recall having been given tooth cleaning instruction or advice about gum care from their dentist.

There is clearly greater interest in using personal oral health products than was demonstrated in previous decades and these improving trends appear to be stronger than those apparent for reported dental attendance. There appears to be very little evidence to assume that the public, even those who admit only attending the dentist when

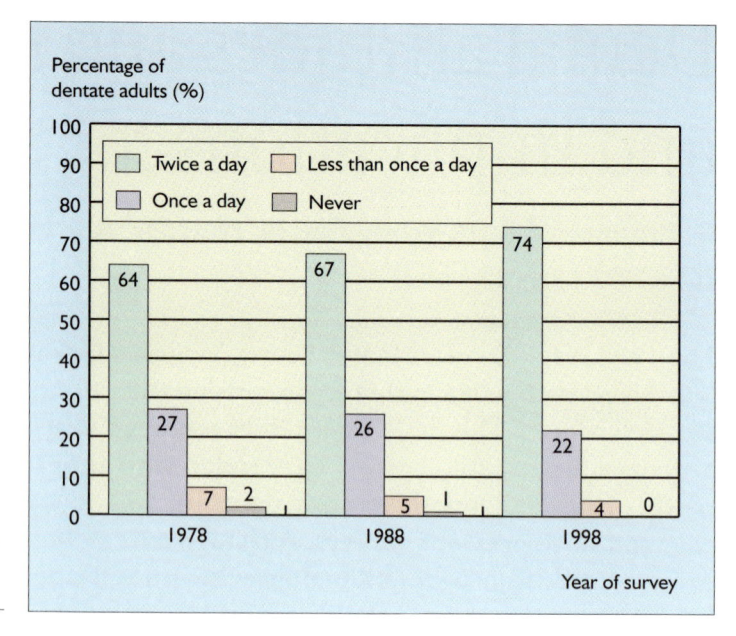

Fig. 2 Frequency of tooth cleaning in the UK, 1978–1998

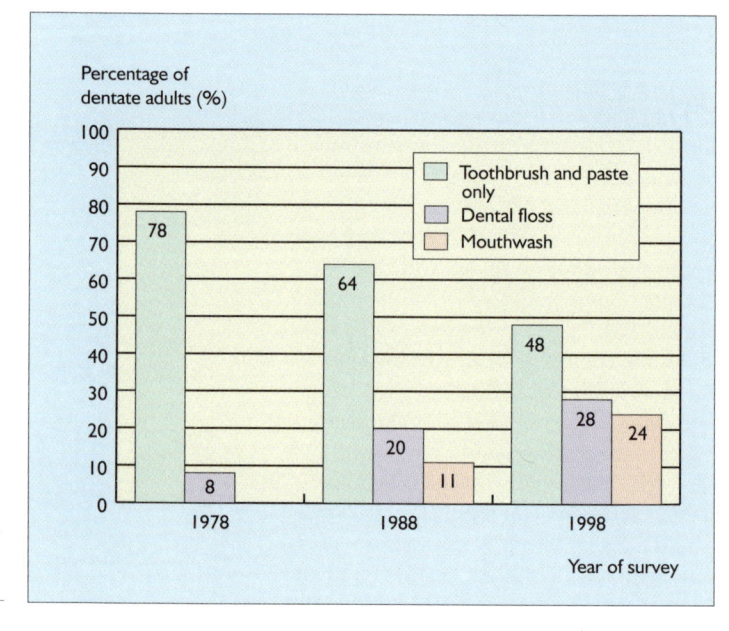

Fig. 3 Use of oral hygiene products in the UK, 1978–1998

> **In brief**
> - Attitudes towards dental health are more positive than in previous surveys of adult dental health
> - Basic oral health messages are now well embedded in the folklore of the UK community
> - Seventy-nine per cent of adults said they would rather have an aching back tooth filled than extracted
> - Sixty-one per cent of adults with no denture experience were very upset at the thought of wearing full dentures

in trouble, are apathetic about their dental health and their dental progress.

What treatment might people prefer for their teeth?

Since the inception of the studies, respondents have been asked whether they would prefer their front or back teeth to be extracted or restored and positive trends toward restoration have been observed over the decades. Responses to treatment preferences for front teeth could be regarded as having both oral health and aesthetic considerations, since extraction of front teeth imply adverse consequences for appearance. Conversely treatment of back teeth are less likely to be subject to these considerations and changes in attitude toward the treatment of posterior teeth might be considered as relating more closely to more positive attitudes to oral health.

Dental attitudes and behaviours

Table 1: Treatment preferences of dentate adults by social class and country

Treatment preferences	Social class of the head of the household			Country				All dentate adults
	I, II, IIINM	IIIM	IV, V	England	Wales	Scotland	Northern Ireland	
	%	%	%	%	%	%	%	%
Would prefer an aching back tooth to be:								
taken out	13	26	34	20	30	24	24	21
filled	87	74	66	80	70	76	76	79
Would prefer a front tooth to be:								
taken out	5	11	14	8	14	8	8	8
crowned	95	89	86	92	86	92	92	92
Would prefer a back tooth to be:								
taken out	25	39	43	31	31	39	39	32
crowned	75	61	57	69	69	61	61	68
Base	2483	1431	915	3010	682	953	636	5281

The questions that were asked relating to treatment preferences give an indication of attitudes towards retention of natural teeth. For front teeth, unsurprisingly, over 90% of adults said that they would prefer a crown to avoid an extraction, as this would almost inevitably lead to wearing of a denture for aesthetic considerations.

For back teeth just over three-quarters of adults overall (79%) said they would rather have an aching back tooth filled rather than extracted. Although this represented only a small increase since the 1988 survey, it was a 15% increase since 1978. When given the choice of a crown rather than an extraction, 68% of adults said they would prefer a crown.

Clear differences were apparent between adults from different social classes; those from non-manual backgrounds were more likely to prefer a restorative option for a tooth compared with adults from manual and unskilled backgrounds. For example, three-quarters of adults from non-manual backgrounds would rather have an aching back tooth crowned rather than extracted compared with 61% of those from manual and 57% of those from unskilled backgrounds (Table 1).

There were also differences between adults from different countries; those from England were least likely to prefer an extraction rather than a filling for an aching back tooth whereas adults from Wales were most likely to prefer an extraction. Those from Northern Ireland and Scotland were the most likely to prefer extraction to a crown for a back tooth.

Despite the fact that there are still some individuals who would prefer extractions to restorative treatment, clearly this is now a minority view and this again indicates a growing awareness of the UK population to the possibility of retaining their teeth for life.

How satisfied are people with the appearance of their teeth?

Aesthetic considerations can be a major oral health incentive to adults, particularly now that people are less likely to suffer high levels of disease and discomfort. With this in mind, questions relating to how satisfied people feel with their teeth have been included in the adult studies. Twenty-seven per cent of dentate adults indicated that they were dissatisfied with the appearance of their teeth, a similar proportion to 1988, (Fig. 4). Thirty-six per cent of those who indicated that they only attended when in trouble were dissatisfied with the appearance of their teeth compared with only 23% of those who attended regularly. It would appear that 36% either do not feel strongly enough about this situation to consider it worth a visit to the dentist or they do not believe that the dentist can improve their appearance.

Table 2 shows the reasons given for dissatisfaction with dental appearance. The most common reason given was colour, followed by tooth alignment, spaces and broken teeth.

A guide to the UK adult dental health survey 1998

Fig. 4 Dissatisfaction with appearance of teeth or dentures in the UK, 1988–1998

Percentage of dentate adults (%)

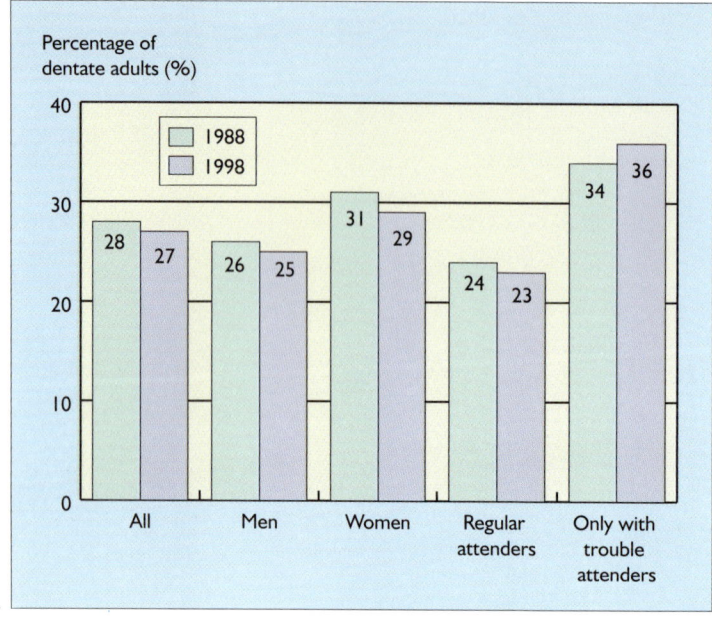

	1988	1998
All	28	27
Men	26	25
Women	31	29
Regular attenders	24	23
Only with trouble attenders	34	36

What unsolicited opinions did people offer?

Thirty-one per cent (1,797) of adults participating in the interview responded to the opportunity to add further comments. Those who responded tended to be from the middle age-bands, from England and Wales, particularly the south of England and from the higher socio-economic groups. Although the comments varied widely certain themes and trends could be captured, showing an emphasis on cost concerns, a perceived drift of primary dental care away from the NHS and difficulty in accessing an NHS dentist. It remains unclear from these data whether these problems exist more among the groups outlined or whether these particular groups are more likely to add unsolicited comments.

How do people feel about having dentures?

Most adults still perceived that denture wearing was a possibility for them in the future. We have seen throughout the series of reports that adults increasingly wish to keep their own teeth and would be upset if they were to require dentures. In 1998, 28% of adults were seen to still be reliant on complete or partial dentures. Since 1968, the perception of having to wear complete dentures as an inevitable feature of ageing has changed. It is now more likely for adults to consider the wearing of full dentures as stigmatic. In 1998, 61% of adults who had no experience of wearing dentures were very upset at the thought of wearing complete dentures. However, only 27% were very upset at the thought of wearing partial dentures. These proportions did not alter dramatically when compared by reported regularity of attendance. A slightly greater proportion of those who reported regular attendance indicated that they would be very upset at having to wear full dentures (30%) when compared with those who only attended when in trouble (21%). This difference was not statistically significant however and cannot be confirmed to be the main reason why people regularly attend the dentist.

Table 2   Reason for dissatisfaction with appearance of teeth, 1988–1998

Dentate adults dissatisfied with appearance of teeth (or dentures) — United Kingdom

Reason for dissatisfaction	1988	1998
	%	%
Colour of teeth	38	48
Crooked/slanting/protruding/irregular teeth	36	34
Gaps/spaces in mouth	13	18
Fillings/colour of fillings	11	10
Decayed teeth	7	5
Size/shape of teeth	6	9
Broken/chipped teeth	5	11
Need filling	0	3
Other	1	8
Base	956	1416

Percentages may add to more than 100% as respondents could give more than one answer.
Base for 1988 as presented in the 1998 report

Dental attitudes and behaviours

Implications for the future

The data presented in the adult dental health surveys, over three decades of reporting, indicate a steadily improving approach toward more positive dental health attitudes. In particular there is a strong indication that adults increasingly wish to retain their natural teeth and are prepared to undertake certain procedures that have been recommended to them by the dental profession and others. The most important indicator must be the increase in people who would prefer their aching back tooth to be restored rather than extracted. These data are strengthened by the growing reported increase in toothbrushing and use of dental floss and mouthrinses.

There is an underlying concern apparent in the data demonstrating that those who have greater oral health needs and those from the more deprived households are still lagging behind in terms of their oral health attitudes. This is not surprising, but it continues to disappoint those who have worked toward equity in oral health. Increased use of oral health aids may be related to advice from the dentist, to advertisements in glossy magazines or to availability of oral health materials in the higher priced supermarkets and high street pharmacies. It is most likely to be a combination of these factors and it remains a major issue that one group of the population are not experiencing similar benefits to the others. It might be concluded that adult oral health continues to be a measure of social exclusion and as such this must be remedied.

This article has been refereed under the British Dental Journal reviewing process. Full details of sample numbers can be found in the survey report. We would like to acknowledge the work of Alison Walker, Maureen Kelly and other staff of the Office for National Statistics. This work was undertaken by a consortium comprising the Office for National Statistics and the Dental Schools of the Universities of Birmingham, Dundee, Newcastle and Wales who received funding from the United Kingdom Health Departments; the views expressed in this publication are those of the authors and not necessarily those of the Health Departments nor of the other members of the consortium.

1. Nuttall N M, Bradnock G, White D A, Morris J, Nunn J H. *Dental attendance in 1998 and implications for the future.* Br Dent J 2001; **190**: 122-127.
2. Steele J S, Treasure E T, Pitts N B, Morris A J, Bradnock G. *Total tooth loss in the United kingdom in 1998 and implications for the future.* Br Dent J 2000; **189**: 598-603.
3. Kelly M, Steele J, Nuttall N, Bradnock G, Morris J, Nunn J, Pine C, Pitt N, Treasure E, White D. *Adult dental health survey: Oral health in the United Kingdom 1998.* London, The Stationary Office 2000.

The oral cleanliness and periodontal health of UK adults in 1998

A. J. Morris,[1] J. Steele,[2] and D. A. White,[3]

Periodontal disease continues to be a major concern for dentists and patients. This paper reports the findings of the 1998 UK Adult Dental Health survey in relation to plaque, calculus, periodontal pocketing and loss of attachment. It is apparent from this study that moderate periodontal disease remains commonplace amongst UK adults and that the associated risk factors of plaque and calculus are in abundance, even amongst those who profess to be motivated about their oral health and attend the dentist regularly. The continued high prevalence of disease needs to be seen in the context of the far larger number of people who are now potentially at some risk, particularly in the older age groups, because of improvements in tooth retention. However, the cumulative effect of disease means that control of the periodontal diseases, even mild and slowly progressing disease, will be a key issue if large numbers of teeth are to be retained into old age. If that level of control is to be achieved we need a widespread improvement in our management of the disease, particularly in our ability to improve the oral cleanliness of the UK population.

As one of the two major oral conditions affecting the adult population, it is important to measure the prevalence of periodontal diseases as part of a national survey of oral health. Periodontal diseases have been recorded in some format in all of the previous surveys of adult dental health in the UK, but continuity has been a problem because of changing concepts of the disease and how best to record and report it.[1] The methodology adopted in the 1998 study[2] was designed to provide a 'best fit' between conflicting requirements. On one hand to allow comparison with previous studies,[3] whilst on the other to reflect contemporary concepts and reflect the new patterns of disease resulting from increasing retention of natural teeth late into life.

A major consideration in adopting criteria was that they had to be as simple as possible. A large number of examiners required training and calibration and, with the examination taking place in the home rather than a surgery, the lighting, seating position and limited range of instruments made accurate recording of periodontal data a challenge. Even with very simple indices, there are still difficulties for survey examiners.[4,5] Plaque and calculus can be difficult to see against a similarly coloured tooth surface, while measuring both periodontal pockets and loss of attachment simultaneously is a tiring and back straining process for the examiner. The pattern of the diseases is also complicated and makes reporting the data difficult, there being no simple indicator of disease experience and activity. An additional complicating factor is the very high prevalence of disease and its dependence on tooth retention so that describing these patterns in a way that is useful and meaningful to the profession is as great a challenge as collecting the data in the first place.

The variables recorded were visible plaque, calculus, pocketing and loss of attachment. Calculus has been measured consistently since the 1968 survey. Plaque on the other hand has not been recorded in its own right since the 1968 survey, though in 1978 debris, which included plaque, was recorded. A measurement of the extent of plaque was re-introduced in 1998 not only because of its fundamental role in the periodontal diseases, but also because it gives us an indication of the effectiveness of tooth cleaning, potentially the most important self-administered preventive dental intervention available for adults. Loss of attachment was also quantified for the first time in this survey. This is a more robust measure of historical disease experience than pocketing alone since it records movement of the point of attachment of the periodontal tissues from the normal position around the neck of the tooth. This is probably a more meaningful measure of the impact of disease in the growing population of dentate older adults than pocketing alone. Pocketing continued to be recorded separately, since it is still an important prognostic indicator and may also indicate a treatment need. The 1998 study reported very deep pockets (greater than 8.5 mm) for the first time so that more severe cases could be identified. The equipment was restricted to light, mirror and CPITN-C probe. A full description of the methodology and criteria appears in the main report.[2]

All dentate respondents who agreed to an oral examination were asked a series of screening questions to identify any whose health might theoretically be put at risk by the examination. Of the 3,817 respondents examined, 300 (8%) were excluded on these grounds. This is likely to be a higher proportion than in the previous 1988 study, particularly for older respondents, because of ethical committee advice to exclude additional respondents with prosthetic joints as well as those with any suspicion of cardiac

[1]*Lecturer in Dental Public Health, School of Dentistry, The University of Birmingham;* [2]*Senior Lecturer in Restorative Dentistry, University of Newcastle upon Tyne;* [3]*Lecturer in Dental Public Health and Behavioural Science, School of Dentistry, The University of Birmingham*
*Correspondence to: A. J. Morris, Dental Public Health, School of Dentistry, St. Chads Queensway, Birmingham, B4 6NN
REFEREED PAPER
Received 02.05.01; Accepted 07.06.01
© *British Dental Journal* 2001; **191:** 186–192

A guide to the UK adult dental health survey 1998

valve defects who would have been excluded by the 1988 criteria. A further ten respondents declined the periodontal examination, having agreed to the rest of the examination, presumably because it involved probing soft tissue.

The prevalence of the various conditions can be described at mouth (subject) as well as tooth level. The latter is important where the prevalence is high at the mouth level since it is a more discriminating measure of differences between groups of subjects. Loss of attachment is reported in similar categories as pocketing, with 3.5 mm as the threshold for diagnosis since it was measured using the bands on the CPITN-C probe.

Results

Plaque and calculus

Plaque was recorded only if it could be seen with the naked eye, without running an instrument along the gingival margin. Consequently, there had to be quite a large accumulation of plaque on the tooth before it was coded as present. In normal circumstances, such a deposit would take a number of days to accumulate. Calculus was recorded both visually and with the help of a CPITN probe.

The prevalence of recorded plaque was high; nearly three-quarters (72%) of subjects examined had visible plaque on at least one tooth and there were only relatively small differences between groups of respondents (Table 1, Fig. 1). There were also only relatively small differences between population subgroups in the mean proportion of respondents' teeth that had visible plaque on the surface. Perhaps surprisingly, the groups with the highest proportion of teeth affected by plaque also tended to have fewer teeth to clean. Overall, the mean proportion of teeth with plaque rose from 30% in the 25–34 year age group to 44% in the 65 years and over group. Those respondents who reported that they attended the dentist for regular check-ups were less likely to have plaque (68%) than other respondents (72–80%), and had a smaller proportion of teeth affected (29% compared to 43% in people who attend only with pain). In other words, they had cleaner mouths but although this difference is statistically significant, it is not great in practical terms.

One of the more interesting findings was that the participants who cleaned their teeth immediately before the examination (6%) still had, on average, plaque on almost one-third of their teeth; little different from those who chose not to. In this context, it is perhaps no great surprise that, although participants who reported cleaning their teeth twice daily or more were less likely to have visible plaque (69%) than people who cleaned once daily or less (79–87%), there were still over two-thirds of these self-declared regular brushers who had visible plaque deposits.

Around three-quarters (73%) of subjects had calculus present on at least one tooth and there was an increase in the mouth prevalence with age, from 61% amongst 16–24 year olds to 83% amongst those aged 65 years and over. The tooth prevalence of calculus showed a similar variation with age though the range was greater. There was a

Table 1   Visible plaque and calculus in dentate adults

Proportion of:	adults with visible plaque	teeth with visible plaque	adults with calculus	teeth with calculus
All dentate adults	72	33	73	23
Age				
16–24	72	34	61	15
25–34	70	30	71	21
35–44	72	32	74	25
45–54	69	32	77	26
55–64	75	37	77	28
65 and over	78	44	83	33
Gender				
Men	76	38	76	26
Women	68	29	70	20
Social class				
I, II, IIINM	70	30	71	21
IIIM	75	36	75	25
IV, V	78	40	76	27
Reported dental attendance				
Regular check up	68	29	68	19
Occasional check up	72	32	75	21
Only with symptoms	80	43	82	32
Reported frequency of tooth cleaning				
Never/less than once a day	87	55	78	38
Once a day	79	41	79	29
Twice a day	69	30	70	21
More than twice a day	69	31	73	21

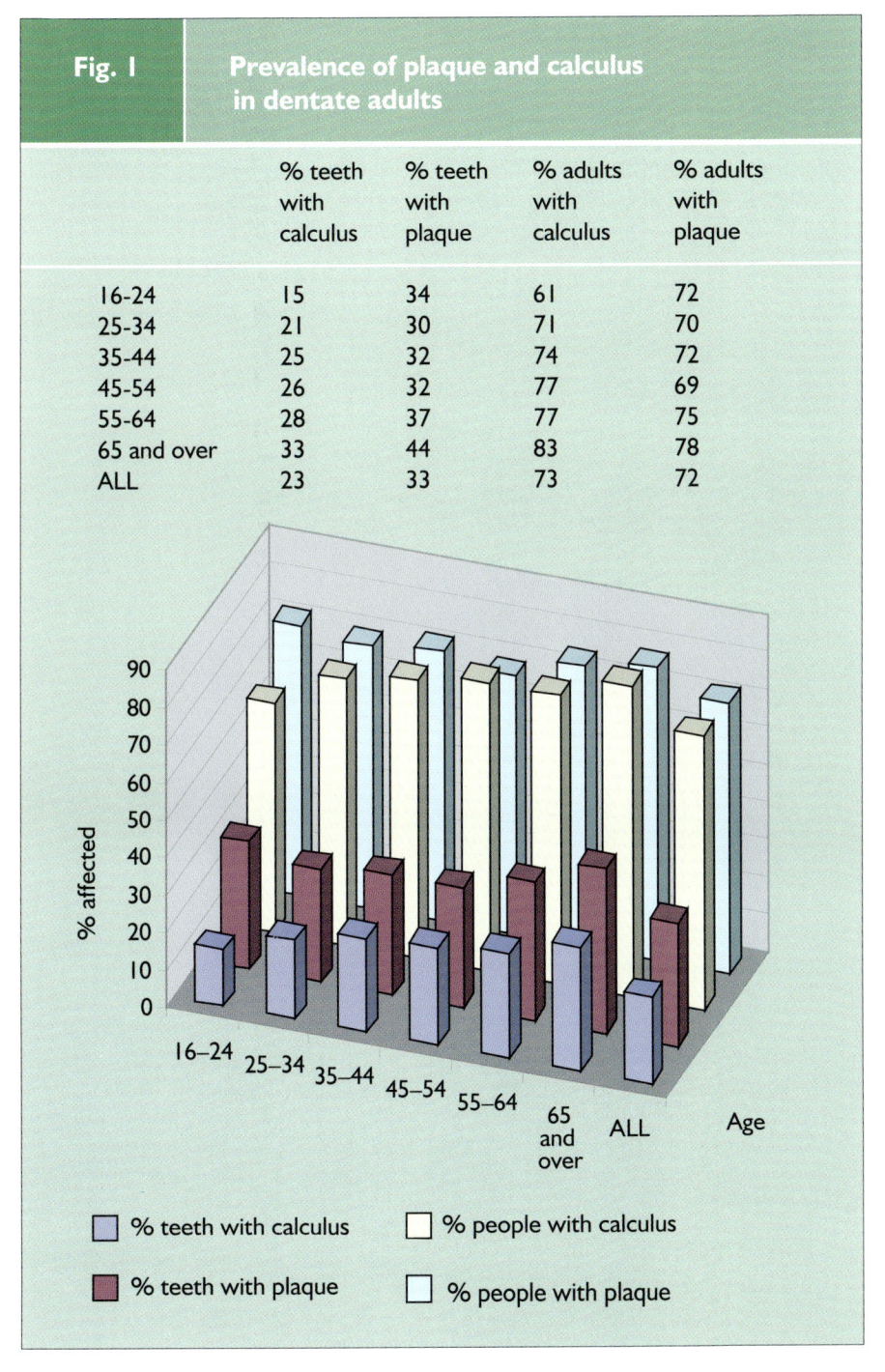

Oral cleanliness and periodontal health

Fig. 1 — Prevalence of plaque and calculus in dentate adults

Age	% teeth with calculus	% teeth with plaque	% adults with calculus	% adults with plaque
16-24	15	34	61	72
25-34	21	30	71	70
35-44	25	32	74	72
45-54	26	32	77	69
55-64	28	37	77	75
65 and over	33	44	83	78
ALL	23	33	73	72

the examination had calculus, this was compared with 84% of respondents who reported that their last dental visit had been between one and five years previously. At the level of the teeth, 19% of teeth in the former group had calculus present compared with 28% in the latter. As expected, the distribution of calculus at different sites in the mouth was not even; only 11% had calculus present on a maxillary canine or incisor (upper central sextant) compared with 67% who had calculus present on the corresponding mandibular teeth (lower central sextant). This reflects what dentists often report seeing in their patients, calculus affecting lower front teeth because of their close proximity to the submandibular salivary ducts, whilst upper front teeth are often the cleanest teeth in the mouth because people often take most care with them.

Pocketing

Pocketing was recorded in three categories based on the familiar CPI scoring system. Over half (54%) of subjects examined had moderate pocketing or worse (greater than 3.5 mm) on at least one tooth (Table 2, Fig. 2). There was a marked increase in the mouth prevalence with age from 34% amongst the 16–24 year age group to 67% amongst those aged 65 years and over, even though the latter age group had on average far fewer teeth and may well have had periodontally affected teeth extracted in the past. The mouth prevalence of deeper pocketing (greater than 5.5 mm) was 5% in all subjects and also varied by age; less than 1% in the 16–24 year age group compared with 15% in the 65 years and over age group. The mouth prevalence of very deep pocketing (greater than 8.5 mm) was only 1% amongst all dentate respondents. Differences in the prevalence of pocketing between groups of subjects other than by age were relatively small.

The site-specific nature of the experience of periodontal disease was reflected in the relatively low tooth prevalence compared with the mouth prevalence; 12% of teeth examined had pocketing greater than 3.5 mm compared with 54% of mouths. The tooth prevalence of pocketing greater than 3.5 mm varied greatly with age; there was

two-fold increase in the proportion of teeth with calculus with increasing age, from 15% in 16–24 year olds to 33% in those aged 65 years and over, reflecting the findings for plaque. Amongst those who reported that they attended the dentist regularly for check ups, 19% of teeth had calculus compared with 32% of teeth in those who reported that they only attended the dentist when troubled by symptoms. The mouth and tooth prevalence of calculus also varied by reported time since last dental visit; 68% of participants who reported that their last dental visit had been less than a year before

A guide to the UK adult dental health survey 1998

nearly a five-fold difference between those aged 16–24 year age group (5%) and the 65 years and over age group (23%). Differences between social classes and by reported attendance pattern remained small, though those who reported visiting the dentist within the last year were almost half as likely to have moderate pockets as those who reported not having visited the dentist in the last five years (11% compared with 20%). An unexpected finding was the slight increase in the mouth and tooth prevalence of pocketing greater than 3.5 mm between those who reported that they cleaned twice a day and those who reported more frequent cleaning. Though the numbers were small, this may be because some of those who were cleaning more than twice a day were doing so because they were aware of having established disease and were making strenuous efforts to remove plaque.

Loss of attachment

Loss of attachment was measured from the level of the cemento-enamel junction to the base of the pocket. The millimetre categories used were the same as those for pocketing. In total, 43% of dentate respondents examined had loss of attachment greater than 3.5 mm on at least one tooth and there was an increase in the mouth prevalence with age from 14% amongst the 16–24 year age group to 85% amongst the 65 years and over age group (Table 3). The mouth prevalence of loss of attachment greater than 3.5 mm was lower than the mouth prevalence of pocketing greater than 3.5 mm in the younger age groups and higher in the 55–64 year and 65 years and over age groups. This reflects higher levels of gingival recession in older adults and 'false pocketing' resulting from mild gingival enlargement without attachment loss in younger people. Recession was likely to be a very common feature in the older age groups and reflect a lifetime's disease history. Because of this, loss of attachment, which takes account of recession, indicates the real threat to the tooth from loss of periodontal support more accurately than pocketing in older adults. The mouth prevalence of loss of attachment greater than 5.5 mm was 8% in all dentate respondents examined and also varied with age; less than 0.5% in the 16–24 year age group compared with 31% in the 65 years and over age group. As with pocketing, the tooth prevalence of loss of attachment was far lower than the mouth prevalence; 10% of teeth examined had loss of attachment of greater than 3.5 mm compared with 43% of mouths. The tooth prevalence of loss of attachment of greater than 3.5 mm varied greatly with age, being 2% in the 16–24 year age group compared with 30% in the 65 years and over age group. This suggests that much of the pocketing reported in younger age groups was 'false pocketing' resulting from enlarged gingivae rather than attachment loss. Differences between social classes and in reported attendance pattern were small.

Severe disease

Moderate disease is widespread, but it is those with severe disease who cause the greatest of clinical problems and these are the individuals who are at greatest risk of tooth loss. Although they occupy only a

Table 2	Pocketing			
Proportion of dentate adults with:	No pocketing above 3.5 mm	Pocketing greater than 3.5 mm	Pocketing greater than 5.5 mm	Pocketing greater than 8.5 mm
All dentate adults	46	54	5	1
Age:				
16–24	66	34	1	0
25–34	53	47	2	0
35–44	41	59	5	0
45–54	39	61	6	1
55–64	38	62	9	1
65 and over	33	67	15	4
Gender				
Men	43	57	6	1
Women	49	51	5	0
Social class of head of household				
I, II, IIINM	48	52	6	1
IIINM	44	56	5	1
IV, V	44	57	7	1
Reported dental attendance				
Regular check up	48	52	5	1
Occasional check up	45	56	4	1
Only with symptoms	43	57	6	1
Reported frequency of tooth cleaning				
Never/less than once a day	38	62	7	0
Once a day	42	58	6	1
Twice a day	49	51	5	1
More than twice a day	44	56	6	0

Oral cleanliness and periodontal health

Fig. 2 Prevalence of pocketing

Proportion of dentate adults with:	No pocketing above 3.5 mm	Pocketing 4 mm–5.5 mm	Pocketing 6 mm–8.5 mm	Pocketing greater than 8.5 mm
16–24	66	33	1	0
25–34	53	45	2	0
35–44	41	54	5	0
45–54	39	55	5	1
55–64	38	53	8	1
65 and over	33	52	11	4
ALL	46	49	4	1

ferer of severe disease will have a very high proportion of teeth affected by pockets at some level, but typically there will be relatively few which are severely affected at any one time and there will usually be a reasonable proportion of relatively unaffected teeth (Fig. 3). Loss of attachment of over 5.5 mm affects more people in the population than pocketing of the same depth, particularly amongst older adults, but the numbers and proportions of teeth affected in those with relatively advanced loss of attachment is strikingly similar to that for deep pocketing, and the distribution of affected teeth is similar (Fig. 4). Once again there are a few teeth severely affected, but on a base of teeth which are moderately affected.

The people who are more severely affected are rather difficult to single out or to profile. The social and gender influences appear to be negligible, they do not necessarily have the dirtiest mouths and they are not much more likely to be dental non-attenders. They are, however, likely to be older. Although this may in part be that the measures are of disease experience rather than activity, the increase in the prevalence of deep pockets and extensive loss of attachment later in life is quite dramatic.

Discussion

The data derived from a large survey of this sort are necessarily crude. Only a limited number of variables are recorded and maintaining the accuracy of measurements is difficult. Examiners find it particularly difficult to probe posterior teeth during a home examination, so the prevalence of deep pocketing and loss of attachment is probably under-recorded. Nevertheless, the population sample is large, highly representative of the UK public and the data quality issues described will not greatly affect the differences between age groups or associated with reported attendance behaviour, nor the relative lack of differences between social and gender groups. As it is possible that inter-examiner variability could give biased results by geographical region we have avoided any comparison between areas, though there is no particular reason to expect any major effect in this regard either.

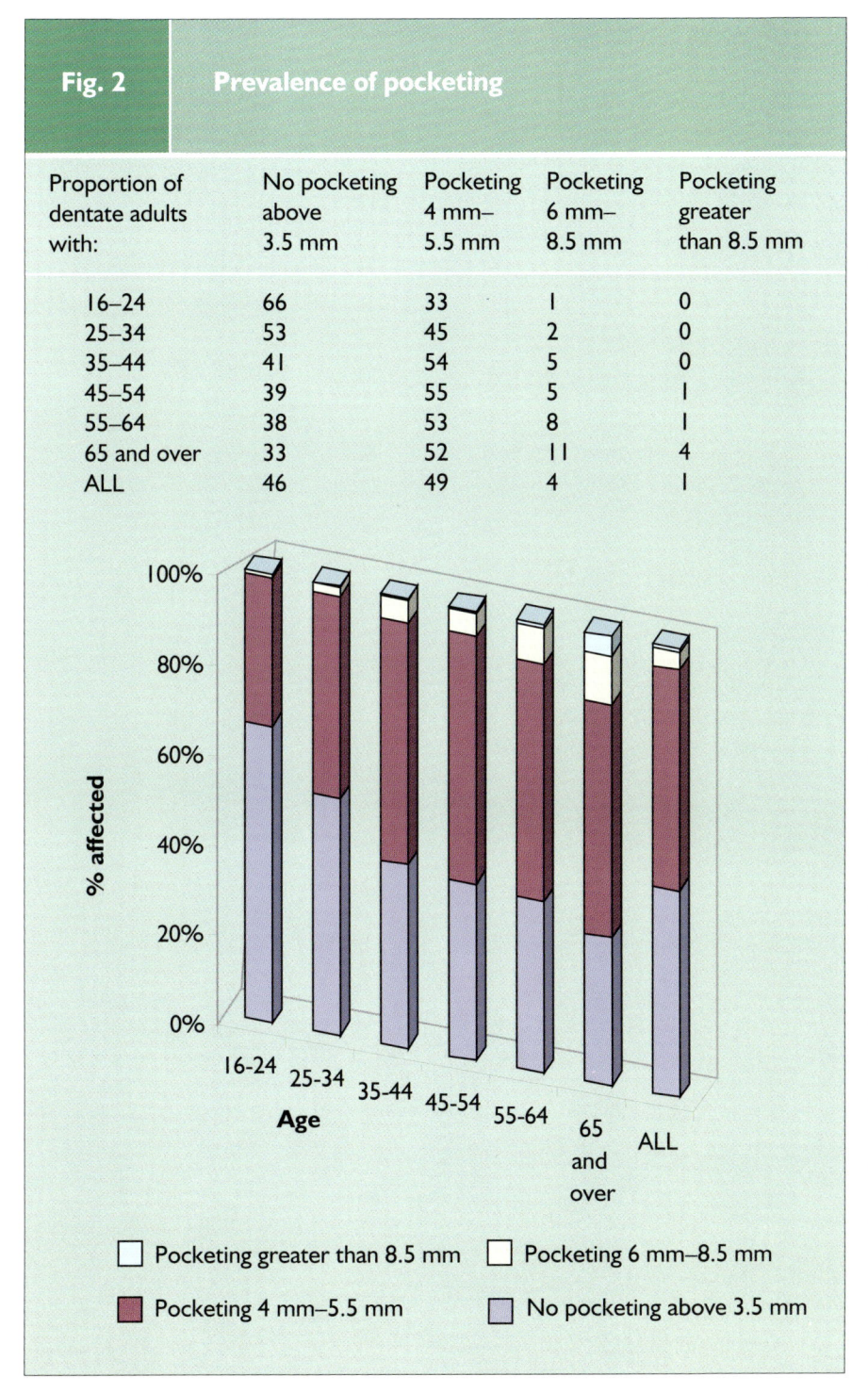

small proportion of the dentate population this group is important, but it is easy to lose sight of them in a mass of population data. Amongst the 5% who have a pocket of over 5.5 mm, they have on average nearly three teeth affected (mean 2.6) by such deep pocketing, whilst they will have around ten of their teeth affected by pocketing which is at least moderate (mean 11.4 teeth, 54% of all teeth). In other words, the average suf-

A guide to the UK adult dental health survey 1998

Table 3	Loss of attachment (LOA)			
Proportion of dentate adults with:	No LOA above 3.5 mm	LOA greater than 3.5 mm	LOA greater than 5.5 mm	LOA greater than 8.5 mm
All dentate adults	57	43	8	2
Age				
1–24	86	14	0	0
25–34	74	26	2	0
35–44	58	42	3	0
45–54	48	52	10	2
55–64	30	70	17	4
65 and over	15	85	31	7
Gender				
Men	54	46	9	2
Women	61	40	7	1
Social class of head of household				
I, II, IIINM	58	42	7	1
IIINM	56	44	9	2
IV, V	53	47	11	2
Reported dental attendance				
Regular check up	57	43	7	2
Occasional check up	61	39	5	0
Only with symptoms	56	44	10	2
Reported frequency of tooth cleaning				
Never/less than once a day	49	51	13	0
Once a day	51	49	11	2
Twice a day	61	39	6	2
More than twice a day	55	45	8	1

When looking at these results, it is worth bearing in mind that only dentate adults and standing teeth contribute to the data. The population experience of disease reported applies only to the 87% of the adult population who have some natural teeth, we know nothing about the former state of the teeth of the edentulous, though technically they are now unaffected. On the other hand, figures reported may well under-estimate historical disease experience, since mouths rendered edentate by disease and extracted teeth in partly dentate mouths (perhaps extracted because of periodontal disease) are both lost to the analysis.

Despite all of these considerations, the results of this study indicate that UK adults have a high prevalence of plaque and calculus on their teeth, with surprisingly little difference between those who report higher levels of dental motivation and those who do not. The regular brushers and reported regular dental attenders did have less plaque than the smaller groups of infrequent brushers and reported non-attenders, but many of the former still had visible plaque on a large proportion of their teeth. The only reasonable conclusion to draw from this is that, despite their apparent efforts, UK adults are not as efficient at plaque control as might be hoped. Oral hygiene is a huge public and personal health issue and improved hygiene could be expected to result in benefits in terms of periodontal disease and dental caries. There is clearly some room for improvement.

Differences in the prevalence of calculus between groups are likely to reflect differences not only in the frequency and effectiveness of tooth cleaning but also the use of dental services for the removal of calculus and the number of teeth present. The effect of reduced numbers of teeth in the mouth on the prevalence of calculus will be limited because the teeth most likely to be retained in those with partially dentate mouths are mandibular canines and incisors, teeth which are more likely to have calculus. This may partly account for the steeper trend in tooth prevalence associated with age. Calculus is however widespread in the UK adult population and the data suggest that dental services do have an impact in the removal of calculus, at least on the removal of visible calculus.

The prevalence of severe pocketing (greater than 5.5 mm) is low overall, but over half the subjects examined had at least one pocket over 3.5 mm present and 12% of teeth were similarly affected. This also increases quite sharply with age, underpinning the need for continued monitoring. The results for loss of attachment indicate a high prevalence of significant loss of attachment in older adults and this would merit closer study in future. Although it is reported in the same way as pocketing, the

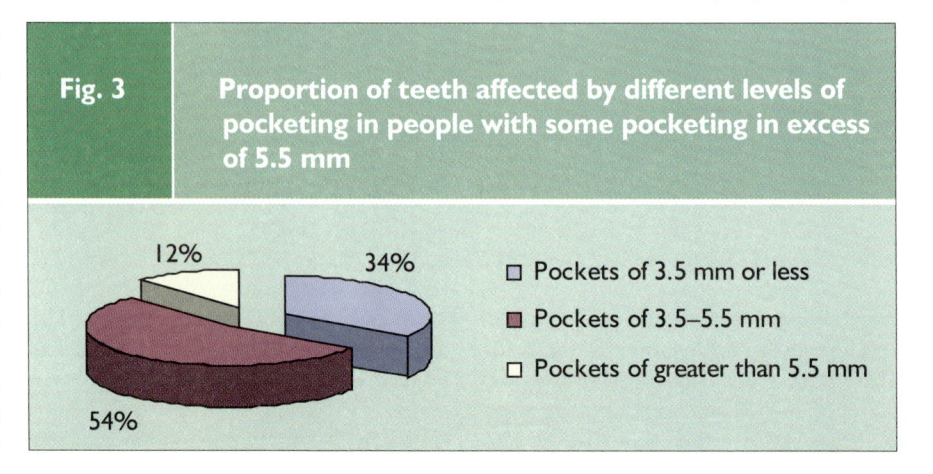

Fig. 3 Proportion of teeth affected by different levels of pocketing in people with some pocketing in excess of 5.5 mm

- 12% — Pockets of 3.5 mm or less
- 34% — Pockets of 3.5–5.5 mm
- 54% — Pockets of greater than 5.5 mm

Fig. 4 Proportion of teeth affected by different levels of loss of attachment (LOA) in people with some LOA in excess of 5.5 mm

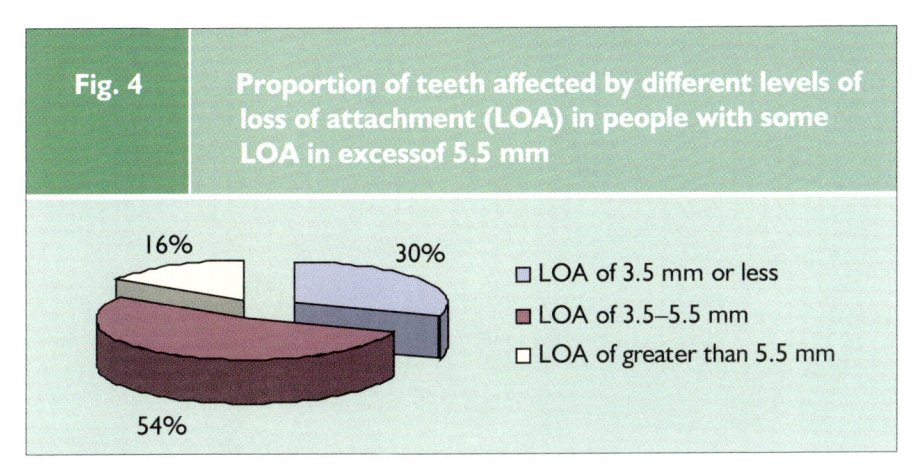

- 16% — LOA of 3.5 mm or less
- 30% — LOA of 3.5–5.5 mm
- 54% — LOA of greater than 5.5 mm

interpretation is a little different; any loss of attachment could be regarded as potentially pathological for the purposes of analysis whereas pocketing is usually only regarded as potentially pathological above about 3.5 mm. Loss of attachment in older adults is often a combination of extensive recession as well as some pocketing. The areas of recession may be where there was a deep pocket in the past, though in some cases we may be looking at creeping recession where deep pocketing was never present. The important point is that attachment loss is generally irreversible and these results show the extent to which attachment is lost over a lifetime where teeth are retained. Moderate and probably slowly progressing levels of disease, which will result in extensive attachment loss and pose a real threat to individual teeth over the course of a lifetime, have affected a significant proportion of the population by the time they reach retirement age. The fact that 85% of dentate people aged 65 years and over have at least some teeth which have seen over 3.5 mm of loss attachment suggests that low grade but slowly destructive disease is the norm.

Differences in the prevalence of pocketing and disease between various population subgroups were generally quite small. Assuming that inherent susceptibility does not vary between study groups, and there is nothing to suggest that it should except possibly with gender, the differences between groups are likely to represent the consequences of a wide range of different factors. These include the frequency and effectiveness of tooth cleaning, smoking and the use of dental services over a long period. The inclusion of tobacco use as a variable may be a valuable addition in future studies, since this is reported to be an important explanatory factor in the development of disease.[7] Neither the reported frequency of oral hygiene practices nor the reported use of dental services seemed to be strongly associated with the prevalence of measurable disease. This finding should be interpreted with caution in view of the complex relationship between health behaviour and disease experience, for example people with identified disease may be making a greater effort to maintain their teeth. Despite these words of caution, it is difficult to escape the suggestion that neither dental services nor attempts at hygiene are having the impact on disease we might hope. Results from elsewhere in the survey suggest that regular dental-attenders benefit in real terms over a lifetime in terms of tooth retention, perhaps by up to as much as five more retained teeth by the age of 65 years.[2] The lack of any major difference in the prevalence of periodontal disease according to reported attendance pattern may suggest that, although it is impossible to be certain of the mechanism, most of this benefit comes through restoration of the teeth, rather than management of periodontal diseases.

Disease of the periodontal tissues continues to be a commonplace finding in the UK, but, being a complex disease to measure, it is difficult to get a real feel for long-term trends. The increased retention of natural teeth presents a particular problem in this regard because as more teeth are retained there are more sites that may be affected by disease, and more people with teeth to be affected. Therefore, we may in part be victims of success on other fronts; even if our management of the disease was improving, the retention of teeth might make it difficult to demonstrate this until we make a considerable impact on the disease. The continued high prevalence needs to be seen in the context of the far larger number of people who are now potentially at some risk, particularly in the older age groups. The cumulative effect of disease means that control of the periodontal diseases, even mild and slowly progressing disease, will be a key issue if large numbers of teeth are to be retained into old age. If that level of control is to be achieved we need a widespread improvement in our management of the disease, but particularly in our ability to improve the oral cleanliness of the majority of the UK population.

We are grateful to the dental examiners, NHS organizers and the Office for National Statistics for their assistance with this study.

1. Chapple I L C. Periodontal disease diagnosis: current status and future developments. *J Dent* 1997; **25**: 3-15.
2. Kelly M, Steele J, Nuttall N, Bradnock G, Morris J, Nunn J, Pine C, Pitts N, Treasure E, White D. *Adult Dental Health Survey: Oral Health in the United Kingdom 1998.* Walker A, Cooper I, ed. London: The Stationary Office, 2000.
3. Todd J E, Lader D. Adult dental health 1988: United Kingdom. London: HMSO, 1991
4. Mojon P, Chung J-P, Favre P, Budtz-Jörgensen E. Examiner agreement on periodontal indices during dental surveys of elders. *J Clin Periodont* 1996; **23**: 56-59.
5. Fleiss J L, Mann J, Paik M, Goultchin J, Chilton N W. A study of inter- and intra-examiner reliability of pocket depth and attachment level. *J Periodont Res* 1991; **26**: 122-128.
6. Gray P G, Todd J E, Slack G L, Bulman J S. Adult Dental Health in England and Wales in 1968. London: HMSO, 1970.
7. Axelsson P, Paulander J, Lindhe J. Relationship between smoking and dental status in 35-, 50-, 65-, and 75-year-old individuals. *J Clin Periodontol* 1998; **25**: 297-305.

Index

Access to healthcare 40, 44
Age associations
   crowned teeth 15, 25, 27
   dental attendance 37
   dental decay 9-10
   dental disease experience 20
   filled teeth 7, 9, 13-14
      root surface fillings 15
   functional dentition 4-5
   medication-related problems 16-17
   oral hygiene in old age 17
   periodontal disease
      calculus 48-49
      loss of attachment 50
      pocketing 49-50
      severe disease 51
   restorations 7, 9, 15, 25, 27
      distribution/number 16
      implications for GDPs 16-17
   root caries 10-11
   total tooth loss 1, 19
Amalgam fillings 15
Anxiety, dental 40
Attendance, dental 35-40
   age associations 37
   calculus prevelance 49, 52
   crowned teeth relationship 15, 25
   decayed/unsound teeth relationship 9-10, 25
   frequency of visits 37, 38-39
   gender associations 37
   impact of oral health conditions 33
   natural teeth retention relationship 4, 14, 36
   population trends 35, 36-37
   reasons for avoidance 39-40
   'regular' check-ups 37-39, 40
   restorations relationship 14, 15, 25
   tooth condition associations 36
   young people 9-10, 37
Attitudes, dental 41-45
   interview questions 41
   unsolicited opinions 44

Behaviours, dental 41-45
   interview questions 41

Calculus 47, 48-49, 52
Caries 9-10
   cavitated lesions 7, 9, 12
   distribution 9
   management issues 9, 12
   root 10-11, 17
   secondary 14
   visual 7, 9, 12
Clinical examination 7, 13, 47
Complete denture prosthetics 5
Cost of dental treatment 39, 44
   estimates 40
Crowns 13, 15
   age associations 15, 25, 27
   multivariate analysis 24, 25
   treatment preferences 43

Decayed/unsound teeth 8, 9
   dental attendance relationship 25
   multivariate analysis 20, 23, 25
Dental disease experience 7-12
   multivariate analysis 20, 22
   see also Tooth condition
Dentures
   functional limitation 33
   future need for complete prosthetics 5
   overnight wear 42
   patient attitudes 41, 44
Denturists 6
Drug-related conditions 16-17

Education/training, dental 5
   denturists 6
Educational attainment 19
Estimates of treatment cost 40

Fear, dental 39, 40
Filled teeth 13-15
   age associations 13-14
   clinical examination 13
   condition of fillings 14-15
   dental attenders 14
   root surface fillings 15-16
   treatment preferences 43
Final clearance 3
Floss use 42, 45
Fluorides 12, 25
Functional dentition 1, 4
   definition 4
   implications for dental profession 5-6

Gender differences
   dental attendance 37
   filled teeth 14
   tooth loss 1, 2
Geographical variation see Regional differences

Handicapping oral conditions 30, 31, 33, 34
Hygiene, oral 12, 41, 42, 52
   advice from dentist 42
   elderly adults 17

Impact of oral conditions 29-34
   clinical oral status associations 32-33
   dental attendance motivation 33
   denture-wearers 33
   disability 30, 31, 33
   discomfort 30, 31
   functional limitation 30, 31
   handicap 30, 31, 33, 34
   impairment 30
   see also Oral Health Impact Profile (OHIP)
Information about dental care 39, 40

Long-term value of treatment 40
Loss of attachment 47, 48, 50, 51, 52-53

Mouthwash use 42, 45
Multivariate analysis 19-27
   decayed/unsound teeth 20, 23, 25
   dental disease experience 20, 22
   implications for professional practice 25, 27
   natural teeth retention 19-20, 21
   periodontal disease 25, 26, 27
   restorations 24, 25
   sound/untreated teeth 20
   total tooth loss 19, 20

Natural teeth retention 1, 4-5, 9, 15-16
   age associations 1
   attitudes 43, 45
   dental attenders 4, 36
   geographical variation 2-3
   implications for GDPs 16, 17
   multivariate analysis 19-20, 21
   numbers of teeth 4-5
   projections of future trends 3-4
   see also Functional dentition

OHIP-14 31, 33-34
  survey results 31-34
    clinical oral status associations 32-33
    dental attendance 33
    frequency of problems 30
    types of problem 31-32
Oral Health Impact Profile (OHIP) 29-31
  shortened scale *see* OHIP-14
Oral health measures 1
Oral health products use 42, 45

Pain experience 31, 34
Patient involvement in treatment planning 39, 40
Peridontal pocketing 47, 48, 49-50, 51, 52, 53
Periodontal disease 3, 4, 47-53
  calculus 47, 48-49, 52
  clinical examination 47
    exclusions on health grounds 47-48
  loss of attachment 47, 48, 50, 51, 52-53
  multivariate analysis 25, 26, 27
  plaque 12, 47, 48-49, 52
  pocketing 47, 48, 49-50, 51, 52, 53
  severe disease 50-51
  survey data collection 47, 51
Plaque deposits 12, 47, 48-49, 52
Poverty 16

Preventive approaches 27
  middle-aged/older adults 17
Professions complementary to dentistry (PCDs) 9, 11
Prosthetic skills, future need 5-6
Psychological discomfort/disability 31, 32, 34

Regional differences
  dental disease experience 20, 25
  tooth loss 2-3, 19
  treatment preferences 43
Restorations 8, 9, 13-17
  age associations 7, 9, 16-17, 25
  clinical examination 13
  dental attendance associations 25
  failure 14, 15
  implications for GDPs 16-17
  multivariate analysis 24, 25
  treatment preferences 42-43, 45
Root caries 10-11, 17
Root surface fillings 15-16, 17

Satisfaction with dental appearance 41, 42, 43
Sealants 9, 12, 20, 27
Social class associations
  crowned teeth 15
  filled teeth 14
  tooth loss 1-2
  treatment preferences 43
Sound/untreated teeth 7-9

  multivariate analysis 20
Survey methods 1, 7, 13, 19, 29, 35, 47

Tooth condition 7-12
  dental attenders 36
  implications for dental profession 12
Tooth wear 7, 11-12
Toothbrushing 12, 27, 42, 45
  periodontal disease relationship 48, 50, 52
Toothpaste use 42
Total tooth loss 1-6
  age associations 1, 19
  gender differences 1, 2
  management issues 6
  multivariate analysis 19, 20
  patient attitudes 6
  patterns of tooth loss 3
  projections of future trends 3-4
    implications for dental profession 5-6
  reasons for final clearance 3
  regional differences 2-3
  social class associatons 1-2
Treatment planning 39, 40
Treatment preferences 42-43

Unsound fillings 15